GENETICS - RESEARCH AND ISSUES

SEX CHROMOSOMES

NEW RESEARCH

GENETICS - RESEARCH AND ISSUES

Additional books in this series can be found on Nova's website under the Series tab.

Additional E-books in this series can be found on Nova's website under the E-book tab.

MICROBIOLOGY RESEARCH ADVANCES

Additional books in this series can be found on Nova's website under the Series tab.

Additional E-books in this series can be found on Nova's website under the E-book tab.

GENETICS - RESEARCH AND ISSUES

SEX CHROMOSOMES

NEW RESEARCH

MARIO D'AQUINO
AND
VINCENTE STALLONE
EDITORS

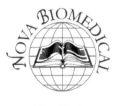

New York

Copyright © 2013 by Nova Science Publishers, Inc.

All rights reserved. No part of this book may be reproduced, stored in a retrieval system or transmitted in any form or by any means: electronic, electrostatic, magnetic, tape, mechanical photocopying, recording or otherwise without the written permission of the Publisher.

For permission to use material from this book please contact us:
Telephone 631-231-7269; Fax 631-231-8175
Web Site: http://www.novapublishers.com

NOTICE TO THE READER

The Publisher has taken reasonable care in the preparation of this book, but makes no expressed or implied warranty of any kind and assumes no responsibility for any errors or omissions. No liability is assumed for incidental or consequential damages in connection with or arising out of information contained in this book. The Publisher shall not be liable for any special, consequential, or exemplary damages resulting, in whole or in part, from the readers' use of, or reliance upon, this material. Any parts of this book based on government reports are so indicated and copyright is claimed for those parts to the extent applicable to compilations of such works.

Independent verification should be sought for any data, advice or recommendations contained in this book. In addition, no responsibility is assumed by the publisher for any injury and/or damage to persons or property arising from any methods, products, instructions, ideas or otherwise contained in this publication.

This publication is designed to provide accurate and authoritative information with regard to the subject matter covered herein. It is sold with the clear understanding that the Publisher is not engaged in rendering legal or any other professional services. If legal or any other expert assistance is required, the services of a competent person should be sought. FROM A DECLARATION OF PARTICIPANTS JOINTLY ADOPTED BY A COMMITTEE OF THE AMERICAN BAR ASSOCIATION AND A COMMITTEE OF PUBLISHERS.

Additional color graphics may be available in the e-book version of this book.

Library of Congress Cataloging-in-Publication Data

ISBN: 978-1-62417-143-7

Library of Congress Control Number: 2012949963

Published by Nova Science Publishers, Inc. † New York

Contents

Preface		vii
Chapter I	The Evolution of Mammalian X Chromosomes and X Chromosome Inactivation *Claudia L. Rodríguez Delgado and Janine E. Deakin*	1
Chapter II	Role of Sex Chromosomes in Mammalian Female Fertility *Asma Amleh, Bao-Zeng Xu and Teruko Taketo*	53
Chapter III	The Fate of the Y Chromosome *Asato Kuroiwa*	87
Chapter IV	The Role of Y Chromosome Genes on Tumor Development Risk in Disgenetic Gonads *Monica Vannucci Nunes Lipay and Bianca Bianco*	109
Chapter V	Deletion of Amelogenin Y-Locus: State of the Art in Gender Determination *Luciana Caenazzo and Pamela Tozzo*	125
Chapter VI	Non-invasive Prenatal Diagnosis for Fetal Sex Determination *Aggeliki Kolialexi, Georgia Tounta, Danay Mavreli, Ariadni Mavrou and Nikolas Papantoniou*	139

| **Chapter VII** | Application of X Chromosomal STR Polymorphisms to Individual Identification
Jian Tie and Seisaku Uchigasaki | **151** |

Index **163**

Preface

In this book, the authors present new research in the study of sex chromosomes. Topics discussed in this compilation include the evolution of mammalian X chromosomes and X chromosome inactivation; the role of sex chromosomes in mammalian female fertility; the fate of the Y chromosome; the role of Y chromosome genes on tumor development risk in disgenetic gonads; deletion of amelogenin Y-locus; non-invasive prenatal diagnosis for fetal sex determination; and application of X chromosomal STR polymorphisms to individual identification.

Chapter I - For many years it was thought that the X chromosome in all three major lineages of mammals (monotremes, marsupials and eutherians) had a shared evolutionary history. However, monotreme and marsupial genome projects and the employment of molecular cytogenetic techniques have enabled the evolutionary history of mammalian X chromosomes to be more accurately traced. This research revealed that monotremes have a complex sex chromosome system consisting of multiple X chromosomes that share no homology to the X chromosome of therian (marsupial and eutherian) mammals. Therian sex chromosomes arose from a pair of autosomes with a subsequent addition to the X chromosome having occurred in the eutherian lineage.

The evolution of mammalian sex chromosomes has led to large, gene-rich X chromosomes and smaller, gene-poor Y chromosomes, which is thought to create an imbalance in transcriptional output between the X chromosome and autosomes in males that requires dosage compensation. This hypothesis has only been thoroughly interrogated since the advent of microarray and RNA-sequencing technologies but the findings of these studies remain controversial. However, it is more generally accepted that the dosage imbalance for X-borne genes between the sexes requires some form of compensation; otherwise females would be expressing twice as much of an X-linked gene as their male counterparts. Compensation for this imbalance is deemed essential, as an extra copy of autosomal genes is usually deleterious. In eutherian mammals, this is achieved by transcriptionally silencing one X chromosome in female somatic cells. Fifty years of research has uncovered many of the features of this remarkable epigenetic phenomenon. However, research into X chromosome inactivation in marsupials and monotremes has lagged far behind that of their eutherian counterparts, largely due to the limited knowledge of genic content of their X chromosomes. Fortunately, genome sequencing of the platypus and several marsupial genomes has alleviated this problem and enabled such research to forge ahead at a great pace. This has led to a number of seminal findings and new hypotheses regarding the evolution of X chromosome inactivation.

Chapter II - Oogenesis takes place in the presence of two X-chromosomes in normal mammalian development. While the second X-chromosome is inactivated in all somatic cells, it is reactivated in the female germ cells prior to the onset of meiosis and remains active in the oocyte. The importance of this exception to the X-dosage-compensation rule is understandable but not formally proven. In this review, we discuss the fertility of females carrying atypical sex chromosomes, namely XO and XY. We will briefly touch on human cases, but mainly focus on mouse models. Our laboratory has been studying the mechanism of infertility in the B6.Y^{TIR} sex-reversed female mouse, which carries a single X-chromosome and an intact Y-chromosome. We review the findings from our study of this particular mouse model, with emphasis on the behaviour of sex chromosomes during the meiotic progression in the XY oocyte and the consequent ooplasmic defects leading to a failure in the second meiotic division.

Chapter III - The mammalian X and Y chromosomes were originally a homologous pair of chromosomes. The accumulation of deleterious mutations and the subsequent inactivation and loss of Y-linked genes could have led to the genetic degeneration of the Y chromosome over evolutionary time, approximately 300 million years (Myr). In modern humans, only approximately 45 Y-linked genes remain. Most of these have acquired functions that are essential for maleness, for example, sex determination or spermatogenesis. It has been proposed that the loss of human Y-linked genes is inexorable and might lead to the extinction of the entire species because of the active role that this chromosome plays in male function. The contrary opinion suggests that the remaining Y-linked genes are strictly conserved through purifying selection. Recent comparative genomic analysis among the Y-chromosome sequences of primates, human, chimpanzee, and rhesus macaque, showed a high level of conservation of human Y-linked genes, at least over the past 25 Myr of the human lineage. However, rodents include very interesting species in which complete loss of the Y chromosome has occurred. Two species of Ryukyu spiny rat and one species of mole vole have an XO/XO sex chromosome constitution due to absence of the Y chromosome. Furthermore, in these species, a key mammalian sex-determining gene, *SRY*, was also lost upon disappearance of the Y chromosome. These XO species show us that loss of the Y chromosome would not lead to the extinction of humans, and there are several processes of Y evolution in our future.

Chapter IV - The presence of Y-chromosome material in patients with dysgenetic gonads increases the risk of gonadal tumors, especially gonadoblastoma (GB). In 1987, Page hypothesized that there is a locus, termed GBY (gonadoblastoma on the Y chromosome), which predisposes the dysgenetic gonads to developing such *in situ* tumors. Studies have been suggested that the testis-specific protein Y encoded (TSPY) repeated gene is the putative region for this oncogenic locus, and could potentially be involved in other human cancers. Hildenbrand et al. studied a patient with TS and a 45,X/46,X,mar karyotype who developed unilateral gonadoblastoma. Cytogenetic and molecular studies confirmed that the marker was derived from a Y chromosome. The authors investigated the gonadal material by immunohistochemistry for the expression of the *TSPY* gene, and the results revealed a high level of TSPY protein expression. However, one of the Y sequences most frequently used in Turner Syndrome (TS) patients screening is the *SRY* gene, because of its localization and its important role in the signaling cascade of sex determining events.

It is already well established that the presence of Y-chromosome material in patients with dysgenetic gonads increases the risk of gonadal tumors, such as gonadoblastoma and dysgerminoma, or of nontumoral androgen-producing lesions. This confers clinical importance to the detection of the Y-chromosome mosaicism in TS.

Screening for Y-chromosome specific sequences is important in the follow-up of TS patients, considering that it is correlated to the proven risk of gonadal tumors development. Thus, the early detection of such events could be of great importance to preventing of gonadal tumor development in TS patients.

The *SRY* gene plays a pivotal role in the signaling chain that occurs during embryonic development, functioning as an activator and also being regulated by several genes. Moreover, it is of fundamental importance in cell differentiation and, consequently, in the determination of the gonadal microenvironment, which starts interacting in the presence of androgens. This way, genes that perform in sex differentiation and development would have an altered expression in the dysgenetic gonads of TS patients, possibily implying in gonadal tumorigenesis. Significant difference in the dysgenetic and controls gonads regarding the expression of genes *OCT4*, *SRY*, and *TSPY* in both gonads of a case characterized by temporal exposure of dysgenetic gonads to the Y-chromosome sequences. This fact could lead to neoplastic development as a result of accumulated modifications in the gonadal microenvironment, especially under the hormonal activity that characterizes the pubertal period, even in the absence of histopathologic abnormalities of the gonads.

Chapter V - Accurate gender determination is widely used and it is crucial in many scientific disciplines, especially in profiling for DNA databasing, forensic casework (e.g., identifying the gender of biological material in stains of unknown origin), analysis of archeological specimens, preimplantation/prenatal diagnosis and post-natal diagnosis (e.g., X-linked diseases or children with ambiguous genitals). Today, molecular techniques, also based on length variation in the X–Y homologous amelogenin gene (AMELX and AMELY), are used for sex determination. In humans, the amelogenin gene is a single copy gene located on Xp22.1–Xp22.3 and Yp11.2 and it is sufficiently conserved, so the simultaneous detection of the X and Y alleles using polymerase chain reaction can lead to gender determination. There is a size difference of 6 bp between the X and the Y genes in the most widely used PCR primer set. The presence of two amplified products indicates a male genotype, while a single amplicon implies a female genotype. Several studies, published since 1998, have shown that normal males may be typed as females with this test because the amelogenin gender test may not always be concordant with true male gender: AMELY deletions may result in no amplification product and normal males being typed as female with the test (negative male).

To date literature data have supported that the null allele is the result of a larger deletion on the short arm of the Y chromosome and that this occurs in different percentages in different population groups. Considering the consequences of the result obtained using only the amelogenin marker and the potential related interpretation difficulties, the gender misinterpretation may be troublesome in some cases, both in clinical practice and forensic caseworks.

Different strategies have been proposed to solve this misinterpretation, such as the use of additional markers to resolve the possible occurrence of

AMEY deletion. In this paper we propose a review of the incidence in failures of gender testing among different populations and the different strategies proposed in literature in case of doubt regarding the presence of deleted AME in the DNA profile.

Chapter VI - Clinical indications for fetal sex determination include risk of X-linked disorders, a family history of conditions associated with ambiguous development of external genitalia and some fetal ultrasound findings. It is usually performed in the first trimester from fetal material obtained through CVS and is associated with an approximately 1% risk of miscarriage. Ultrasound fetal sex determination is often performed after 11 weeks of gestation.

Diagnosis of fetal sex was one of the earliest developed tests for non invasive prenatal diagnosis (NIPD) from the 7th week of gestation using cell free fetal DNA (cffDNA) circulating in maternal plasma. The majority of reported studies are based on quantitative real-time PCR (RT-qPCR) analysis of the SRY gene, achieving sensitivities of 90–100%, with an extremely low incidence of false positive results. False negative results are usually due to failure of amplification of the SRY gene in male fetuses caused by undetectable levels of cffDNA in maternal plasma. A gender independent fetal marker is therefore necessary to verify the presence of fetal DNA sequences. Female fetuses are not detected directly, but by the absence of Y chromosome specific sequences.

Fetal sex determination by cffDNA analysis is currently performed clinically in many centers in order to avoid conventional invasive testing in pregnant women at risk for X-linked and endocrinal disorder.

Chapter VII - The human DNA markers most commonly utilized in individual identification are autosomal short tandem repeat (STR), followed by Y-chromosome STRs and mitochondrial DNA. X-chromosomal short tandem repeat (X-STR) loci may efficiently complement autosomal markers in paternity testing, especially in deficient paternity cases with female offspring, and in kinship analysis involving large and incomplete pedigrees. X-STR loci are located on the non-recombining region of the X chromosome and are inherited as a block of linked haplotypes. Due to its unique inheritance pattern, the X chromosome is a potential candidate for forensic and human identity testing applications. Currently, more than 40 X-STRs have been established as forensic markers, and a large number of population data have been published. X-STR haplotyping can be of particular help in kinship testing in deficient paternity cases where a DNA sample from one of the parents is not available for testing. The ideal technique for X-STR typing is multiplex PCR, because as the number of polymorphic loci examined increases, the probability of identical alleles being present in two different individuals decreases. Multiplex systems have been developed in order to apply X-STRs efficiently for paternity testing. In view of the wide application of these markers, several X-STRs multiplex PCR systems have been validated for individual identification, which include four to thirty markers. Multiplex with greater number of markers are being developed to obtain a high degree of discrimination. Samples from a mass disaster site or from a crime scene exposed to environment are often not only highly degraded but also in very scarce quantities, making it difficult for scientists to perform multiple PCR analyses. Analysis of degraded DNA samples using mini X-STR multiplex systems will offer high efficacy for personal identification.

In: Sex Chromosomes: New Research ISBN: 978-1-62417-143-7
Editors: M. D'Aquino and V. Stallone © 2013 Nova Science Publishers, Inc.

Chapter I

The Evolution of Mammalian X Chromosomes and X Chromosome Inactivation

Claudia L. Rodríguez Delgado and Janine E. Deakin
Division of Evolution, Ecology and Genetics, Research School of Biology,
The Australian National University, Canberra, Australia

Abstract

For many years it was thought that the X chromosome in all three major lineages of mammals (monotremes, marsupials and eutherians) had a shared evolutionary history. However, monotreme and marsupial genome projects and the employment of molecular cytogenetic techniques have enabled the evolutionary history of mammalian X chromosomes to be more accurately traced. This research revealed that monotremes have a complex sex chromosome system consisting of multiple X chromosomes that share no homology to the X chromosome of therian (marsupial and eutherian) mammals. Therian sex chromosomes arose from a pair of autosomes with a subsequent addition to the X chromosome having occurred in the eutherian lineage.

The evolution of mammalian sex chromosomes has led to large, gene-rich X chromosomes and smaller, gene-poor Y chromosomes, which is thought to create an imbalance in transcriptional output between the X chromosome and autosomes in males that requires dosage compensation.

This hypothesis has only been thoroughly interrogated since the advent of microarray and RNA-sequencing technologies but the findings of these studies remain controversial. However, it is more generally accepted that the dosage imbalance for X-borne genes between the sexes requires some form of compensation; otherwise females would be expressing twice as much of an X-linked gene as their male counterparts. Compensation for this imbalance is deemed essential, as an extra copy of autosomal genes is usually deleterious.

In eutherian mammals, this is achieved by transcriptionally silencing one X chromosome in female somatic cells. Fifty years of research has uncovered many of the features of this remarkable epigenetic phenomenon. However, research into X chromosome inactivation in marsupials and monotremes has lagged far behind that of their eutherian counterparts, largely due to the limited knowledge of genic content of their X chromosomes.

Fortunately, genome sequencing of the platypus and several marsupial genomes has alleviated this problem and enabled such research to forge ahead at a great pace. This has led to a number of seminal findings and new hypotheses regarding the evolution of X chromosome inactivation.

Introduction

Sex can be determined in a variety of ways, ranging from environmental sex determination (ESD) mostly seen in invertebrates and some reptiles, to genetic sex determination (GSD). In mammals and birds, sex is typically determined in a GSD fashion, were the locus that triggers sex determination is located on the sex chromosomes.

Mammals have an XX/XY system, where males are the heterogametic sex, whereas birds follow a ZZ/ZW system, in which females are the heterogametic sex. Although the systems are superficially similar, with a gene rich X and Z chromosome and often highly degraded Y and W chromosomes, comparative analyses have revealed that sex chromosomes have evolved multiple times during evolution and any resemblance is the results of convergent evolution [1].

Mammals are divided into three main extant groups: Eutheria ('placental') mammals, Metatheria (marsupials) and Prototheria (monotremes). Eutherian mammals are divided into four superordinal clades: Euarchontoglires, Laurasiatheria, Xenarthra and Afrotheria, the latter representing the most basal clade.

Eutherian mammals diverged from marsupials 148 million years ago (MYA). Together, Eutheria and Metatheria encompass the Theria clade, which diverged from monotreme mammals 166 MYA [2] (Figure 1A). Features common to all mammals are that they possess fur and produce milk to feed their young but it is their mode of reproduction that easily distinguishes the three lineages (Figure 1B).

Eutherian mammals are characterised by prolonged *in utero* development in the presence of an invasive placenta. The most commonly studied representative species are *Homo sapiens* (human) and *Mus musculus* (mouse). In evolutionary studies, the value of including a representative from the Afrotheria has made *Loxodonta africana* (African elephant) an important species. Marsupials give birth to altricial young, which typically develop in a pouch or marsupium. In this lineage, evolution has placed a greater emphasis on *ex utero* development and a more complex lactation system when compared to their eutherian counterparts.

Most studies on marsupial sex chromosomes have been performed in the American marsupial model opossum (*Monodelphis domestica*), which belongs to the Ameridelphia clade, and the Australian marsupial tammar wallaby (*Macropus eugenii*), representative of the Australidelphia (Figure 1A), both of which have had their genomes sequenced [3, 4]. The most intriguing lineage is perhaps the monotremes, as they exhibit both mammalian and reptilian features. These mammals lay eggs yet their young are fed milk produced by mammary glands. There are only two extant genera, Platypoda, represented by one species of platypus (*Ornithorhynchus anatinus*), and Tachyglossa, comprising four species of echidna [5] (Figure 1A). The platypus genome has been sequenced, making it the model monotreme species for sex chromosome studies [6].

Comparisons between sex chromosomes of all three major lineages of mammals have made it possible to trace the evolutionary history of their sex chromosomes. This was initially achieved by painstakingly mapping individual genes found on the human X and determining their location in other distantly related species.

The advent of genome sequencing has greatly accelerated the pace of progress in this field. Likewise, advances in gene expression technology, such as microarray and RNA-seq analysis, have facilitated research into the resulting consequences of sex chromosome evolution on gene expression. It is these findings that we will focus on in this chapter.

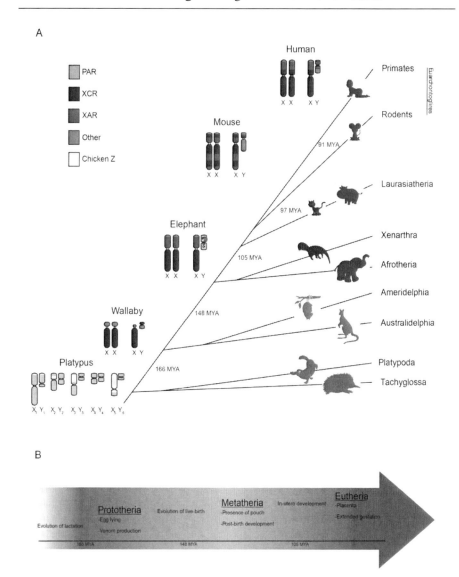

Figure 1. A) Phylogeny showing the three extant mammalian clades, estimated time of divergence [2] and schematic representation of the sex chromosomes in model organisms from each clade. The eutherian clade is represented in *purple*, metatherian (marsupials) in *green* and prototheria (monotremes) in *blue*. 'Other' (in *grey*) may refer to autosomal homology (in platypus), heterochromatin or unknown. B) Physical features unique to a particular clade or shared within clades. Colours as above.

Sex Chromosome Evolution

It is now widely accepted that sex chromosomes evolved from an autosomal pair as first observed by Muller in 1914 [7], after the proto-Y (or W) chromosome acquired a sex-determining locus (testis determining factor - TDF). To ensure that this acquired locus, together with sexually antagonistic genes within close proximity remain in phase, recombination was suppressed, leading to accumulation of deletions and beneficial mutations in the non-recombining region. This resulted in progressive degradation of the proto-Y. Deleterious mutations accumulate faster because of the hemizygous nature of the Y chromosome. Accumulation of mutations could have been driven by further evolutionary forces: background selection, where weak advantageous mutations are eradicated due to co-existence with strong deleterious mutations; Mueller's ratchet where genetic-drift aggravates Y-degeneration; the Hill-Robertson effect where loss of nearby weakly selected beneficial mutations and deleterious mutations occurs due to their proximity; and hitchhiking in which a deleterious mutation is fixed following selection for a beneficial variant [reviewed in 8]. In absence of recombination, the proto-Y genes started to differentiate from the X partner, leading to subfunctionalization and acquisition of novel functions on the Y. In addition, amplification events originating multiple Y gene copies also led to neofunctionalization [9].

Rapid degradation of the proto-Y chromosome primarily by deletion events and accumulation of repetitive elements resulted in the small, gene-poor, heterochromatic Y we see today, which typically bears male-beneficial genes. Comparative genomics studies along the vertebrate lineage support the hypothesis of an autosomal ancestor, as sex chromosomes from different lineages are orthologous to autosomes in the others. Comparative genomics has even revealed some surprises in the origin of mammalian sex chromosomes.

Evolution of the Therian X Chromosome

In uncovering the evolutionary origin of mammalian sex chromosomes it makes sense to start by comparing the gene content of the gene-rich X chromosome between distantly related species, as the X would more closely resemble the autosome from which the X chromosome originated. For many decades, performing these types of comparisons between eutherian species such as human and mouse, and representative marsupials and monotremes was painstakingly slow and, as later uncovered upon the availability of genome sequence data, was not always accurate. Sequence data changed our understanding of the evolution of mammalian sex chromosomes.

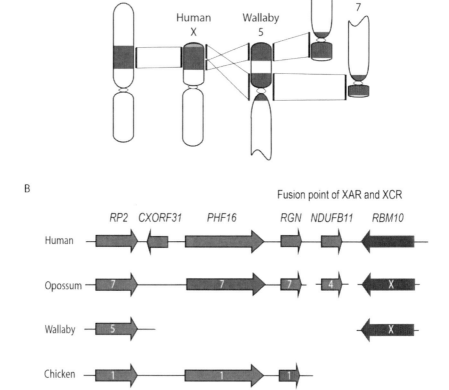

Figure 2. A) A region (XAR) was added to the therian X chromosome soon after marsupial/eutherians divergence. The XAR, depicted in *red* on the human X, is autosomal in marsupials and found as two conserved blocks in the tammar wallaby and opossum. This region is found on chicken chromosome 1 as one conserved block. B) Narrowing down the fusion point of the XAR (genes in *red*) to the XCR (genes shown in *blue*) to the region between *RGN* and *RBM10* on the human X chromosome. Only *RP2* and *RMB10* have been assigned to chromosomes in the wallaby [10]. *RBM10* is absent from the chicken genome assembly.

Early work using comparative gene mapping and chromosome painting between human and tammar wallaby showed homology of the tammar wallaby X chromosome to the long arm of the human X (Xq) and the pericentric region of the short arm (Xp) [11, 12]. This conserved region in therian mammals, referred to as the X conserved region (XCR), is at least 147 million years old. An additional region, known as the X added region (XAR) was added to the X soon after divergence of marsupials and eutherians, as it is autosomal in marsupials, mapping to chromosome 5 in the tammar wallaby (Figure 2A) [10, 13-15] but is present on the elephant X chromosome.

The 155Mb human X chromosome, representing 5% of the haploid human genome, has since been completely sequenced [16], and found to contain ~1,500 genes. The opossum X chromosome is smaller at just ~80Mb (the tammar wallaby X is larger due to a large heterochromatic short arm), accounting for 3% of the haploid genome and harbouring ~513 genes (Ensembl 68). By comparing the gene content of the human X with that of the sequenced opossum X, it was possible to elucidate the precise border where the addition of the XAR occurred. The fusion point for this addition corresponds to human Xp11.23, and lies between the genes *RGN* (found on opossum chromosome 7) and *RMB10* (found on the opossum X chromosome) (Figure 2B) [3]. Gene mapping in the tammar wallaby has also narrowed down the border of the XCR and XAR to this same region [10]. Interestingly, the elephant centromere is positioned in the region corresponding to human Xp11.23, suggesting that the XAR fused to the ancestral therian X by means of a Robertsonian fusion sometime after their divergence from marsupials 147 MYA and before the radiation of the eutherian lineage ~105 MYA [17].

Gene Structure of Therian X Chromosomes

The X chromosome gene content and arrangement is well conserved among eutherians with conserved synteny observed between human, cat [18], cattle [19], horse [20] and elephant [17]. Interestingly, although rodent gene content is conserved, several rearrangements have disrupted gene order [21] (Figure 3). Gene content is also conserved between marsupials and eutherians, with at least 322 orthologues identified between opossum and human XCR [22]. However, gene arrangement is not conserved between these two lineages [3, 10] or even among marsupials (Figure 3). For instance, a comparison of the opossum and human X chromosomes identified at least 26 breakpoints [3]. Based on the mapping of 47 tammar wallaby and 15 Tasmanian devil X-borne genes, gene order was found to be scrambled between opossum, tammar wallaby [10] and Tasmanian devil [23].

Conversely, the genes from the eutherian XAR region show a much higher degree of conservation in gene order between eutherians and marsupials, occurring as two conserved blocks on the tammar wallaby and opossum autosomes (Figure 2A). Both blocks are found on tammar wallaby chromosome 5 [10], but distributed on two different chromosomes in the opossum; the short arm and pericentric region of chromosome 4 and the pericentric region of chromosome 7 [3].

The XCR contains 659 and 442 protein-coding genes in human and opossum, respectively (based on Ensembl 68). The human and mouse X chromosomes have been augmented by amplification of testis-specific genes families [24, 25], and expansion of the cancer-testis antigen gene family in primates [26]. These amplified multicopy families are contained within large inverted repeats especially on three regions of the human X (Xp11, Xq22 and Xq28) [25] and have been reported to account for 12% of the mouse X chromosome [24]. Moreover, genes involved in early (but not late) spermatogenesis are enriched on the human and mouse X chromosomes [27-29].

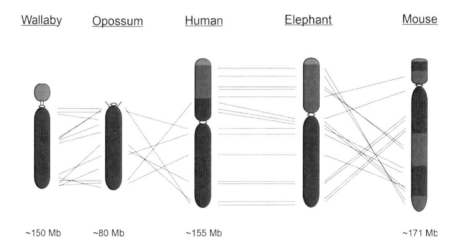

Figure 3. Schematic representation of the X chromosome. The XCR is coloured in *blue*, XAR in *red* and heterochromatic region in *grey*. Lines present the location of orthologous genes between species, showing numerous rearrangements occurred in marsupials and in mouse X chromosome.

The human and mouse X chromosomes show a bias for genes involved in brain development and reproduction [28, 30, 31]. Ubiquitous expression in brain and testis from a subset of X-linked genes and the observation of recurrent association between X-linked mental retardation (XLMR) conditions and genital trait aberrations and infertility led to the 'brains and balls genes' hypothesis [32]; stating that the same X-linked genes were independently selected for intelligence by sexual selection (where smarter males are selected by females), and for reproduction by natural selection (conferring reproductive advantages to males), thereby explaining their expression in brain and testis. Were these genes independently recruited to the eutherian X followed by sexual selection? In the tammar wallaby, brain-related genes are located in two conserved blocks on the X chromosome as well as tammar chromosome 5 [33]. For instance, the *AKAP4* gene lies on the human XCR and is essential for signal transduction and sperm motility regulation in humans and mouse [34]. In wallaby, it is X-linked and its expression is confined to adult testis, while the product is detected in sperm tail in wallaby and mouse, providing evidence for a conserved role in marsupial and eutherian spermatogenesis [4, 35]. The human XAR *KAL1* gene maps to the wallaby XAR homologous region in chromosome 5, and shares sequence homology, expression patterns and function with its human counterpart, providing evidence for its ancestral role in gametogenesis [36]. A second XCR human gene, *TGIFLX*, is not present in the tammar genome, although its precursor, *TGIF2* maps to chromosome 1 and exhibits similar expression patterns restricted to round spermatids as *TGIFLX* in mouse and human [37]. Besides, expression of three mouse XLMR genes (*ARHGEF6, OPHN1, PAK3*) was tested in chicken, where they are expressed in brain, but testis expression is restricted to mouse [38]. Together, these results suggest that even though the ancestral therian X was already enriched for 'brains and balls' genes, specialization of some X-linked genes occurred later in the eutherian lineage, and further autosomal segments containing spermatogenesis-related genes were conscripted. Thus, the X chromosome appears to retain and recruit sex- and reproduction- related genes, particularly those with male specific function.

A separate process shaping X chromosome gene structure is the silencing of male sex chromosomes during male meiosis, known as meiotic sex chromosome inactivation (MSCI). This silencing occurs during the first mitotic prophase, presumably as a response to unpaired X and Y chromosomes, and this repressed status is maintained in round spermatids through post-meiotic sex chromatin (PMSC). This process is observed in all therian mammals, and is achieved in a similar fashion [39, 40]. Thereby, genes necessary for spermatogenesis (e.g. *PGK, PDHA1, RBMX*) have been exported off the X chromosome onto autosomes through retrotransposition to ensure their expression during meiosis [41, 42]. Recent evidence from mouse microarray and RNA fluorescence in situ hybridization (RNA-FISH) suggests that retrotransposition occurs for genes expressed during meiosis, and that genes expressed after meiosis are retained on the X [24]. Retrotransposition from autosomes to X chromosomes has also been described in human and mouse, as suggested by intron-depleted X-linked genes (e.g. *ATXN3L, YY2*) [43].

Monotreme Sex Chromosomes

Analyses of platypus sex chromosomes provide valuable insights into sex chromosome organization and evolution due to their unique phylogenetic position between reptilian/avian and mammalian lineages. However, determining the evolutionary history of monotreme sex chromosomes was not straightforward, particularly because deciphering which chromosomes represented the sex chromosomes was challenging. Chromosome sorting by flow cytometry followed by chromosome painting ultimately led to the identification of the sex chromosomes in monotremes [44-46].

In platypus and echidnas, sex chromosomes include ten and nine sex chromosomes, respectively. Each of these sex chromosomes differ in size and gene content. In males, the sex chromosomes form a chain during meiosis [47], with one PAR region of X_1 pairing with the homologous region of Y_1, the other end of Y_1 pairs with X_2, and so forth [48]. A translocation from the echidna chromosomes equivalent to platypus Y_5 and Y_3 explains why a Y chromosome has been "lost" from the echidna genome [49].

Even though they are not common, multiple sex-chromosomes systems (bearing less than four sex chromosomes) have been documented in plants and invertebrates, although the monotreme multiple-sex-chromosomes system appears unique in the vertebrate lineage, where meiotic multiples are usually deleterious [47]. In mammals, multiple sex-chromosomes systems usually involve a single X-to-autosome translocation generally resulting in aberrant outcomes. How did monotremes acquire and maintain this complex sex-determining system?

Two models have been proposed to explain the origin of this system: 1) through independent reciprocal translocations from autosomes to sex-chromosomes [45, 48] and 2) by means of Robertsonian fusion between homologous chromosomes following hybridisation of two different populations [50]. The first hypothesis is probably more likely. Chromosome painting between platypus and echidna demonstrate that the sex chromosomes are not identical between them, as only four of the five X chromosomes share homology, with a remaining unique X in each species, implying an early acquisition of the multiple sex-chromosomes system in monotreme evolution with independent sex-to-autosomes translocations after platypus-echidna divergence ~25 MYA [49].

Originally, gene mapping on the largest platypus X chromosome (X_1) with heterologous cDNA probes and using radioactive in situ hybridisation, suggested homology with the eutherian X and therefore, that the therian X was an ancient sex chromosome [51]. The availability of platypus genome sequence made it possible to map many more genes to platypus X chromosomes and showed that none of the X chromosomes had any homology to the human X [52]. However, homology to the chicken Z (human chromosomes 5 and 9) was found largely on X_5 and to a lesser extent on X_1, X_2, and X_3. The platypus X chromosomes also share homology with human chromosomes 2, 3, 5, 6, 8, 9 and 18 [52].

Thus, the X chromosome of therian mammals is much younger than originally thought, meaning that the therian sex chromosomes have therefore evolved at a much faster rate than initially proposed [52].

Pseudoautosomal Regions

The presence of a region of homology at the termini of X and Y chromosomes, the pseudoautosomal region (PAR) where chromosomes pair at male meiosis, provide further evidence to support the autosomal origin of the X and the Y chromosomes. This association is mediated and stabilised through formation of a synaptotemal complex (SC), which precedes recombination, ensuring proper chromosome segregation during the first mitotic division. The PAR has been identified in various eutherian species [54, 55], with a few rodent exceptions like gerbils and voles [56-61], where the mechanism of segregation remains elusive. A second PAR2 has been described exclusively in humans, and it is not required for segregation [16].

Notably, the PAR is absent in the marsupial lineage [62, 63], thus segregation is not regulated by SC formation. Marsupial sex chromosomes undergo a delayed and asynaptic pairing, which is achieved through formation of a dense plate (DP) structure during mid-pachytene phase and shares components of the SC system [64]. Both eutherian and marsupial sex chromosomes associate to nuclear compartments [65-67]. Moreover, marsupial sex chromosomes also are located on the side of the nucleus closer to cytoplasmic compartments [64], suggesting an alternative means of chromosome pairing in marsupials.

In monotremes, sex chromosomes are held together in the meiotic chain through formation of a chiasma within multiple homologous PARs, which are homologous between each chromosome arm, except for the chromosomes at the termini of the chain Xq_1 and Xp_5 [49,52], with most of platypus Xp_1 and Yp_1 representing PAR. The platypus PAR regions undergo recombination during metaphase, and ensure alternate segregation of sex chromosomes into $X_1X_2X_3X_4X_5/Y_1Y_2Y_3Y_4Y_5$ haploid germ cells [45, 48].

MicroRNAs on the X Chromosome

MicroRNAs (miRNAs) are 18-24bp RNAs that regulate posttranscriptional gene expression by pairing to mRNA and triggering degradation or translational repression [68]. While sequence and expression patterns of some miRNAs are evolutionary conserved, emerging sequencing techniques and computational prediction methods have enabled the identification of species- or lineage-specific miRNAs. Correlation between morphological complexity and miRNA expression in vertebrates propose an influence for miRNAs in determining lineage-specific features [69].

Recently, novel X-linked miRNA clusters have been described in a variety of mammalian species. A higher miRNA density in the mammalian (primates, rodents, dow, cow and opossum) X chromosome compared to autosomes has been documented, together with a pattern of faster evolution in the testis-expressed miRNAs [70]. Additionally, Guo et al [70] described higher substitution rates in human and mouse testis-expressed miRNAs, but not in any other tissue. This pattern of testis-expressed miRNA clusters is found on X chromosomes from various mammals. The primate cluster *MIRN506-MIRN514* is testis-specific and has a potential role in spermatogenesis [71]. In rodents, the mirn-743 to mirn465 cluster contains 19 miRNAs that are expressed exclusively in testis [72, 73]. A large miRNA cluster was identified on platypus X_1 chromosome, harbouring at least 92 mature miRNAs where most of them were exclusively expressed in testis [74]. A similar cluster harbouring 39 actual and potential miRNAs spans 102Kb on the opossum X chromosome and diverged into Mdo-miR-1544 and Mdo-miR-1545 families

[75], the former through tandem duplication events and the latter via transposon-mediated duplication process [76]. More recently, a cluster comprising six miRNAs and spanning ~33Kb was characterized exclusively in primates [77], with predicted target genes involved in controlling sperm maturation and male fertility [77]. Most of these clusters have been described as rapidly evolving, probably shaped by the same forces involved in the evolution of X-linked genes, due to the hemizygosity of the X chromosome and positive selection in males.

Mammalian Y Chromosomes

In mammals, degradation of Y chromosome(s) resulted in highly dimorphic sex chromosomes. Contrary to what is seen for the X chromosome, the Y chromosome is highly diverged between species, variable in size, gene order and content, where active genes in one species have become pseudogenes in another. For instance, the primate Y ranges from 24Mb in chimpanzee to 95Mb in mouse, to 60Mb in human, showing its disparity even between these closely related species [78]. The small heterochromatic Y bears ~50 genes in human, which have acquired mostly testis-specific expression and are involved in spermatogenesis [79]. In most marsupial species, the Y is smaller than its eutherian counterpart, representing ~1% of the haploid genome and an estimated size of ~10Mb [80]. Although less studied, and with little information available on gene content, monotreme Y-chromosomes are clearly subject to degradation, as shown by smaller size compared to their X partners [52].

In males, this means that most X-borne genes are without a matching copy on the Y. Even if there is a Y gametologue, it may have a different function to the X gametologue, effectively leaving X-genes present in only one copy in males.

Dosage Compensation

The disparity in X-gene dosage would have caused a two-fold difference in expression ratio between the X and autosomes in males compared to females. It was therefore proposed that the overall expression of mammalian X chromosomes is doubled in both sexes to equalize the transcription imbalance in the heterogametic sex (Ohno's hypothesis) [81, 82]. This process is known as sex chromosome dosage compensation, although this term has also been used to describe balancing of dosage differences between males and females through X chromosome inactivation (XCI). Hereafter, the term dosage compensation will refer to the process of equalizing dosage between X chromosome and autosomes, and should not be confused with the mammalian XCI compensation mechanism between males and females.

Dosage compensation has long been assumed to be a universal feature with supporting evidence documented in a wide variety of organisms including therian mammals (primarily human and mouse), the fruit fly *Drosophila melanogaster* and the nematode worm *Caenorhaditis elegans*. Underlying regulatory strategies are quite variable; in *D.melanogaster* and *C. elegans* they involve chromatin modifications [83], whereas in mammals it is still unknown if compensation is achieved through permanent modifications in DNA sequence from promoter-enhancer regions or by chromatin modifications [84, 85]. Early studies in *Drosophila* suggested an X-wide twofold increase in transcription exclusive to males [86]. A more complex mechanism was described in *C. elegans*, with hypertranscription of the X chromosome in both XO males and XX hermaphrodites, followed by halved expression from both X chromosomes in hermaphrodites to restore diploid levels [87]. A similar process was proposed in mammals, where X chromosomes are upregulated in both sexes and balanced in females by further inactivation of one X chromosome.

Testing Ohno's Hypothesis

The first evidence for X upregulation in mammals was the observation that the chloride channel gene *Clc4*, which is X-linked in mouse species *Mus spretus* but autosomal in laboratory strains, has twice the level of expression in the former compared to the latter [88]. With the advent of microarray technology, comparisons of global transcriptional output between X-linked and autosomal genes became possible. Since dosage compensation allegedly balances X-linked gene transcriptional levels to that of autosomal genes, it can be verified by estimating the ratio between overall X-linked and autosomal gene expression (X:AA); were X:AA ~1 reflects upregulation of the X chromosome and an X:AA ratio of 0.5 is expected when there is no hypertranscription of the X.

Nguyen and Disteche [85] compared the expression levels from several tissues in primates and rodents, reporting an overall average X:AA ratio close to 1 (i.e. 0.94 for human and 1.01 for mouse), with a small but not significant variation amongst tissues. Interestingly, a higher expression was observed in brain tissues (1.43 and 1.18 in human and mouse, respectively) and no upregulation was reported in haploid germ cells [85], where a single autosome is present, thus indicating that dosage compensation also occurs in the germline. In spermatocytes, a low X expression was observed, consistent with X silencing at male meiosis (MSCI). A separate study using time-course data on mouse ES cells and excluding genes with low expression, revealed upregulation of the X prior to differentiation in males and females, with a consistent ratio ~1, accompanied by a progressive inactivation of X-linked genes in one of the two female X chromosomes [89] (Figure 4A).

These results, together with the observation that expression levels are subject to selection [90] were sufficient to accept dosage compensation as an essential mechanism, which must have evolved to counteract the deleterious effects of X-linked genes haploinsufficiency in the heterogametic sex.

It was not until the emergence of RNA-sequencing (RNA-Seq) technique that dosage compensation could be tested in a broader manner even in non-model organisms. In addition, RNA-Seq yields more sensitivity than microarrays [91], as the latter were originally designed to test differential expression of the same genes under different conditions rather than within the same condition or sample. During the last couple of years, various studies based on RNA-Seq data (mostly reanalysis of similar datasets) have returned contradictory results, thus challenging Ohno's hypothesis and questioning the essentiality of global dosage compensation.

In 2010, Xiong et al. [92] provided the first evidence to question global upregulation of the X. The authors compared the performance of RNA-Seq with that of microarray analysis using data from Nguyen and Disteche [85], demonstrating the limitations of microarray data analysis. In addition, they used publicly available data from 12 and three tissues in human and mouse respectively, and calculated an X:AA ~0.5 in most cases, with a smaller ratio observed in mouse ~0.3 [92]. Notably, higher expression levels were reported in brain and testis, consistent with the findings of Nguyen and Disteche [85]. Additionally, the authors compared protein levels from mouse proteomic data and RNA-Seq from the same set of X-linked and autosomal genes, and found consistent lower concentrations for X-linked genes and protein levels than from those of autosomal origin, thereby refuting global X upregulation (Figure 4B).

However, these findings were questioned by a subsequent study, where the authors argued that the apparent lower expression of X-linked genes compared to autosomes could be biased by the gene content of the X chromosome [93]. As previously explained, the X chromosome is enriched in "brains and balls genes", whose expression is exclusive to testis and brain tissues and have no expression in somatic tissues. Deng et al. [93] reanalysed a subset from previous [92] and newly obtained RNA-Seq data, but excluding genes with null or low expression, most of which were multicopy testis-specific genes. The authors compared X:AA ratios in 16 human tissues, and demonstrated that the ratios increased when raising the minimum expression level threshold required for a gene to be included in the analysis, with a ratio increasing from ~0.5 to ~1 for genes with robust expression. A similar pattern was observed in the mouse tissues tested, where the X:AA ratio was dependent on the inclusion or removal of non or low expressed genes. The proportion of non-expressed genes was higher for the X chromosome than for the autosomes, consistent with the tissue-specific expression of "brains and balls" genes [32], with exception of chromosome 21. In fact, the lowest percentage of non-expressed X-linked genes in mouse and human were found in brain and testis; while in somatic tissues, a high proportion of genes with null or low expression corresponded to reproduction related genes [93]. Reanalysis of mouse proteomic data used by Xiong et al. [92] but considering the skewed content of the X, also revealed an X:A median protein ratio ~1.

A different approach, utilising RNA-Seq and chromatin immunoprecipitation with deep sequencing (ChIP-Seq) in mouse embryonic fibroblasts, was followed to verify RNA Polymerase II occupancy and chromatin modifications in the active X to test for signs of upregulation [94]. Higher occupancy of RNA Pol II and histone marks associated to transcription initiation (Pol II-S5P and H3K4me3) and elongation (Pol II-S2P and H3K36me3) [95-97] were observed on the active X, compared to the haploid autosome complement, suggesting that the X is upregulated both at transcription initiation and elongation in a nonlinear fashion. These results are consistent with a higher X chromosome 5' occupancy of Pol II-S5P observed in undifferentiated mouse ES cells with two active X chromosomes [93].

Although previous microarray studies did not take into account the biased gene content of the X chromosome [85], the nature of the technique favours highly expressed genes *per se*. However, the analysis performed by Lin et al. [89] excluded low expressed genes, a practice that was described as "...inappropriate for measuring the absolute value of the X:AA ratio because a higher fraction of lowly expressed genes on X than on autosomes is excluded from the comparison" [92]. These reports were followed by controversial correspondence between the authors of different studies, regarding inclusion and exclusion of underexpressed genes during analysis and its effect on ratio calculations [98-100].

Is there Global Dosage Compensation?

It is now widely accepted that different organisms, such as birds, fish and silkworm, exhibit partial dosage compensation, thereby lacking a global X upregulation mechanism. Furthermore, it has been proposed that dosage compensation only affects dosage-sensitive genes [101], which would explain the incomplete compensation observed in these organisms. However, in mammals the X:AA ratio deviation from 1 (representing absolute compensation between X and autosomes) was attributed to interchromosomal variability [99], or to noise in RNA-Seq data [93]. Hence, a recent study in humans aimed to determine if this deviation could be explained by compensation of only a subset of genes sensitive to dosage differences [102]. Indeed, the authors found that when restricting the dataset to genes encoding proteins involved in complexes (protein-complex genes), the X:AA ratio is not significantly different from 1, especially for those genes involved in complexes encompassing large number of proteins (more than 7) (Figure 4C). The approach followed by Nguyen and Disteche [85] of increasing the threshold for the levels of expression (described above), is in line with these results, as while increasing the threshold, the proportion of protein-complexes genes is also augmented, suggesting that these genes are highly expressed and thus subject to upregulation [102]. Furthermore, a recent study reported consistent results of exclusive upregulation of protein-complexes genes when comparing expression from human and chicken orthologues [103]. The results support partial dosage compensation, affecting exclusively dosage-sensitive genes. However, the authors of the latter study argue that protein-complex genes account for ~5% of the total X-linked genes, denoting that upregulation is not achieved in a global fashion.

The previous studies mainly focused on human and mouse dosage compensation. Two very recent analyses included the two other mammalian lineages (marsupials and monotremes) to test dosage compensation and its evolutionary patterns in the mammalian clade [103, 104]. Contrary to previous analyses, these studies compared the expression ratios for genes on the proto-X chromosome, as Ohno's hypothesis states that dosage compensation arose following Y chromosome decay, thus genes requiring compensation would be those present on the ancestral X (proto-X) while newly acquired genes must remain unaffected. In this sense, a better estimate of X upregulation would be the comparison between current X-linked gene expression levels to proto-X expression levels (represented by one-to-one autosomal orthologues in outgroup species). Independent assessment of X:proto-XX ratios of ~0.5 [103, 104] indicate a lack of global upregulation on the eutherian X (primates and rodents). Different results were reported for marsupials, with one study [104] providing evidence for global upregulation of the marsupial X (X:proto-XX ~0.8) whilst the other refutes this possibility with ratios ranging from ~0.5 to ~0.75 for the different marsupial tissues examined [103]. Interestingly, these results are unaffected by removal of testis-specific genes, which are mainly enriched in the recently acquired region of the X chromosome. The authors proposed that the shift, indicating upregulation of the X previously reported [93, 94, 99, 103], is strongly influenced by the inclusion of the recently acquired genes [104]. Comparisons between male and female overall X expression revealed similar expression levels in therians, denoting effective dosage compensation between the sexes [104], which was unexpected in marsupials as they lack a stable X inactivation system (discussed later in this chapter) [105].

The observations in monotremes (platypus) differ from that of therians. Firstly, a M:F ratio ~0.6 on X_5 and on the non-pseudoautosomal region of X_1 [104] is consistent with previous findings that X chromosome inactivation in platypus females is incomplete [106]. Comparison between current X_5 and proto-X_5 expression levels suggested upregulation of the X chromosome in males but not in females [104]. Alternatively, following up-regulation in both sexes, some form of gene silencing may be decreasing expression from X_5 in females, restoring the proto-X_5 to autosome balance in this sex.

How Important Is Dosage Compensation?

Based on the evidence presented above, the model of global dosage compensation between mammalian sex chromosomes and autosomes proposed by Ohno in 1967 has been revisited. Dosage compensation was originally proposed to accompany sex chromosome differentiation [83]. However, lack of global upregulation in sex chromosomes of various organisms, including chicken [107, 108], platypus [106, 109] and potentially therian mammals [103, 104] indicate that sex chromosome evolution is not dependent on dosage compensation.

An X chromosome-wide dosage compensation mechanism was hypothesised as the genes affected by divergence were all linked and haploinsufficiency would have deleterious effects on the organism. However, Y decay was a gradual process [110, 111], suggesting that differences in gene dosage must have been tolerated through relaxed selection. In addition, if dosage compensation arose in response to Y chromosome degradation, compensation should have been achieved in a gene-by-gene basis rather than through a single upregulation event. Current evidence seems to favour this scenario of local upregulation, potentially affecting only dosage sensitive genes [101].

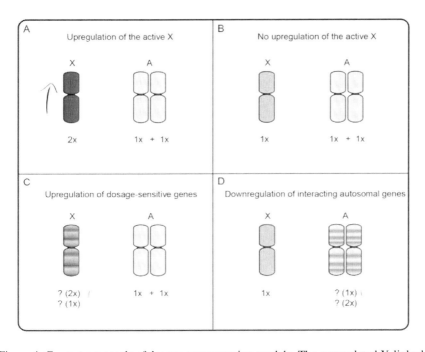

Figure 4. Current proposals of dosage compensation models. The upregulated X-linked genes are coloured in *pink*, non-upregulated X genes in *orange*, autosomal genes in *yellow* and downregulated autosomal genes in *green*. A) Ohno's hypothesis, X chromosome is upregulated (*2x*) to equalize autosomal levels (*2x*). B) There is no dosage compensation between X chromosome (*1x*) and autosomes (*2x*) [92]. C) Only dosage-sensitive genes (protein-complex genes, genes involved in regulatory networks) are upregulated (in *pink, 2x*) while the remaining genes are unaffected (in *orange, 1x*). The number and class of genes upregulated may vary amongst tissues, developmental stages and species (**represented by '?'**) [102]. D) Autosomal genes that directly interact with X-linked genes are downregulated (in *green, 1x*); the remaining genes are unaffected (*yellow, 2x*). '?' represents same as above.

More importantly, the evidence also suggests that dosage compensation is not as critical for development as previously thought [112] and genes seem to be compensated to a level that is sufficient not to compromise the fitness of the organism. In fact, the only viable aneuploidies reported to date are those affecting X chromosomes and chromosome 21, which are the chromosomes bearing the higher proportion of non-expressed genes in somatic cells [93, 113]. Seen from a different perspective, these chromosomes bear the lowest number of dosage sensitive genes [102].

A different model of dosage compensation has been proposed where autosomal genes that directly interact with X-linked genes are downregulated (Figure 4D), diminishing the need for X upregulation [104]. Alternatively, regulation checkpoints could be involved in dosage compensation between sex chromosomes and autosomes; for instance, protein expression could be regulated at different stages in the cell, which would explain why transcriptional regulation is not essential. Another possibility is the need to retain dosage differences for gene function in the sexes (e.g. double versus single dosage required in females and males respectively). A recent hypothesis suggests that dosage differences may have been selected for due to their role in sex-specific functions [114].

Dosage-sensitive genes, as well as genes with critical roles (e.g. protein-complex genes, genes involved in regulatory networks), are targets for dosage compensation. The remaining genes either require a different dosage due to sex-specific functions or are compensated by means of their dosage sensitivity. This theory is consistent with the gene-by-gene basis of X dosage compensation, rather than by a global upregulation of the X. Remarkably, if chromosome-wide upregulation of the X chromosome is ruled out, the role and extent of X chromosome inactivation will need to be re-evaluated.

X Chromosome Inactivation

A consequence of dosage compensation, whether global or piecemeal, is an imbalance in X-borne gene expression between males and females. It is thought that this imbalance needs to be restored to the original transcriptional levels in diploid female somatic cells [110]. Different strategies to counteract this imbalance have been identified in a variety of organisms from *C. elegans* and *D. melanogaster* to eutherians mammals [115].

Based on genetic evidence in female mouse cells, Mary Lyon proposed in 1961 that balancing of X-linked gene expression between females and males in mammals is achieved by silencing one of the two X chromosomes in females, where one of the female X chromosomes is silenced in somatic cells early in embryogenesis and this repressed status is maintained throughout subsequent cell divisions [116]. Since this hypothesis has been proven, it has recently been declared 'Lyon's Law' [117]. This silencing process is known as X-chromosome inactivation (XCI).

Is X Chromosome Inactivation Common to All Mammals?

A shared ancestry of the XCI mechanism might be expected for therian mammals, given the large degree of conservation between the eutherian and marsupial X chromosomes. The lack of homology between monotreme and therian sex chromosomes would suggest that, if monotremes do subscribe to an XCI mechanism, then it would have evolved independently. Hence, the first step to elucidating the evolution of XCI is to determine whether it is observed in all three mammalian lineages.

The Lyon hypothesis was initially based on observations of speckled phenotype in female mice heterozygous for X-linked coat colour mutants [116]. Similar observations made in human population studies on the X-linked gene *G6PD*, with active and deficient erythrocytes in women heterozygous for *G6PD* [118] indicated that approximately the same proportion of cells exhibit maternal (Xm) and paternal (Xp) silencing, leading to the hypothesis that X inactivation in mouse and human is achieved in a random fashion. Evidence to support this hypothesis was provided by an examination of G6PD variants in humans, where only one variant was observed in cultures established from single cells derived from heterozygous females [119]. Observations at the cytogenetic level also supported the idea of an inactive X (Xi), including the presence of a heterochromatic sex chromatin body, referred to as a Barr Body, observed only in female interphase cells [120] and the asynchronous replication of the two X chromosomes during mitosis [121].

The first feature observed to be shared between marsupial and eutherians X chromosomes was the asynchronous replication, which led to the assumption that XCI in marsupials would be similar to that of eutherians [122]. However, early studies in female kangaroos on X chromosome replication timing [123], *PGK* maternal-derived expression [124] and reciprocal crosses of *G6PD-F* electrophoretic phenotype hybrids [125] clearly demonstrated that in marsupials the Xi is always of paternal origin (paternally imprinted). Imprinted X inactivation was confirmed for two other X-linked genes (*GLA* and *HPRT*) and for several different species [reviewed in 126], and was observed in both embryonic and extraembryonic (developing into placenta) tissues in marsupials [127].

Chromatin compaction in the form of a Barr body is observed across all placental mammals [128]. However, although compact chromatin has been observed in opossum embryos [129], it has not been identified in marsupial adult tissues [130]. In platypus, differences in chromatin condensation between three X-chromosomes analysed make it impossible to determine whether it is characteristic of monotreme dosage compensation [131].

Thus, it was concluded that both lineages of therian mammals do subscribe to XCI with at least one common feature but with striking differences as well, most notable the random versus imprinted forms of XCI.

Due to the difficulty in identifying the sex chromosomes, there were virtually no investigations into XCI in monotremes prior to the sequencing of the platypus genome. Early studies examining replication timing of X_1 in fibroblasts found no evidence of asynchronous replication [51, 132], suggesting that monotremes did not inactivate X_1. Data from the platypus genome-sequencing project permitted more thorough examination of X-borne gene expression to be made. A more sophisticated investigation of replication timing for the X-specific regions on three platypus X chromosomes did reveal asynchronous replication [131]. Therefore, asynchronous replication of X chromosomes is a common feature amongst all mammals.

Single nucleotide polymorphisms (SNPs) identified in the DNA of three X-specific genes of the sequenced platypus were analysed by transcript sequencing, showing expression from both alleles. Further real-time PCR analyses demonstrated that the paternal and maternal alleles exhibited equal frequencies of expression, indicating that imprinted XCI does not occur in monotremes [106]. Of course, this did not rule out the occurrence of random XCI.

Expression of X-borne Genes at the Cellular Level

For years, eutherian X inactivation was thought to be complete, affecting the entire X chromosome. Nonetheless, it was discovered that ~15% of human female X-linked genes are expressed from both the Xi and the active X (Xa) in fibroblast [133], and 5% in lymphoblastoid cell lines [134], 'escaping' X inactivation. These escapee genes are mostly located in the eutherian XAR, which probably have not been recruited into the XCI machinery, consistent with the hypothesis of its recent addition. Escapee genes are devoid of chromatin modifications characteristic of the inactive X (explained below) and have a lower expression than their partners on Xa.

Similarly, expression from the Xi was reported in marsupials, with partial inactivation for two genes in some tissues. Early studies from the glycolytic enzyme *PGK-A* showed expression from the paternally derived allele in skeletal and cardiac muscle [135, 136] and in cultured fibroblasts [137] from two Australian marsupials. Further studies from *G6PD* allozymes expression in adult kangaroo tissues and cultured fibroblasts provided similar evidence [138]. Was this lower expression from Xi due to low levels of expression from the Xi in all cells or was it attributed to expression from the Xi in a proportion of cells?

The best way to determine inactivation status of the X chromosomes in females across the three mammalian clades at the cellular level is by looking at expression of genes in individual nuclei. RNA fluorescence *in situ* hybridization (FISH) is a cytogenetic technique, which allows transcript detection from specific loci in individual nuclei. RNA-FISH was performed on three platypus X-chromosomes on female somatic cells [106]. Surprisingly, the results revealed platypus X-chromosomes have a probabilistic mode of expression for X-specific genes, where approximately 50% of fibroblast nuclei expressed an X-borne gene monoallelically and 50% displayed biallelic expression. A more extensive RNA FISH analysis on four platypus X chromosomes confirmed this pattern of expression for more X-linked genes [139]. Consistent with the shared homology between platypus and chicken sex chromosomes, RNA-FISH experiments showed a similar probabilistic mode of expression in chicken fibroblast nuclei. Co-localization of nuclei signals in platypus are consistent with the existence of a single active X-chromosome, and a single X in which genes are prone to inactivation in a proportion of cells [139, 140]. Contrary to what is seen on chicken, the probability of expression of each locus depends on regional coordination of the probability of transcription from adjacent genes, rather than independent probability for each locus [139]. This platypus data raised questions about what was happening in therian mammals.

Similar RNA-FISH based studies across the therian lineage provided valuable information on therian XCI. Stochastic gene inactivation was observed in marsupials and for genes in the XAR in eutherians, similar to the stochastic form of inactivation observed in monotremes, being controlled by the individual probability of expression in each locus rather than downregulation of each locus in all nuclei [141]. However, the pattern of silencing/escape in eutherian XCR, where most of the genes have monoallelic expression [133, 142, 143], is not shared by the marsupial XCR, which in turn has loci with a combination of monoallelic and biallelic expression, demonstrating that orthologous genes in eutherians and marsupials have independent XCI patterns. As discussed in the previous section, evidence for similar X-linked gene expression rates in females and males have been reported [104], contrasting with the stochastic patterns of expression from the marsupial X [105]. On the other hand, current analysis of X upregulation status from the marsupial X is not sufficient to rule out global upregulation of the X [103, 104]. This contrasting evidence perhaps indicates that XCI did not arise as a result of global X upregulation to balance expression levels between the sexes, or perhaps stochastic XCI is a form of dosage compensation itself. However, it must be noted that these analysis were performed in different samples and species (i.e tissue and fibroblast culture in opossum and wallaby respectively) making it difficult to directly compare the association between XCI and dosage compensation in the marsupial lineage. Further analysis on the same samples and species will help to elucidate whether these discrepancies are due to species-specific mechanisms for dosage compensation and XCI.

A striking difference between monotremes and eutherians is silencing in the PAR. While biallelic expression of PAR genes seems to be common in eutherians [141, 144], platypus PAR genes on both X and Y chromosomes have higher rates of inactivation [106]. A more detailed RNA-FISH analysis using nine PAR loci revealed a lower frequency of biallelic expression in all loci, which is not comparable to full biallelic expression in the rest of platypus autosomal genes [139]. Inactivation of PAR genes could be attributed to proximity of these genes to the heterochromatic region, or to upregulation of PAR genes, which needed to be further inactivated to restore basal levels.

The partial/incomplete inactivation seen in birds, monotremes, marsupials and escaper genes on the eutherian X suggest that perhaps female-to-male balancing of X (or Z)-linked genes expression is not as critical as previously thought. It has been proposed that genes subject to equalization could be those with critical roles [145, 146] at the onset of gene pathways or with regulatory functions. Genes under less tight regulation could be those ubiquitously expressed with functions less sensitive to gene dosage, or with multiple regulation steps. Interestingly, most of the partially inactivated genes in marsupials belong to this subset of ubiquitously expressed genes [141]. This could explain tissue-specific escape, where different genes have different roles depending on the tissue, and fits better with the model of gene-by-gene dosage compensation between the X chromosomes and the autosomes.

In conclusion, stochastic X inactivation is observed in marsupials [105], monotremes [109], chicken [139] and escaper genes in eutherians [141]. This evidence together could be interpreted as stochastic X inactivation representing the original state of X inactivation. Although the possibility of an ancient mechanism to control gene expression cannot be ruled out, there appear to be differences in the level of inactivation between the lineages, suggesting potential differences in the inactivation mechanism, which would not be surprising given the lack of homology between monotreme and therian sex chromosomes.

Initiation and Spread of Inactivation in Eutherians

Eutherian X inactivation is initiated at the X inactivation centre (*XIC*) [reviewed in 147]. Originally depicted as a region spanning ~1Mb [148], deletion analysis identified a 80kb region believed to represent the minimum section required to start XCI [149]. The *XIC* contains the X inactive specific transcript (*XIST*), a 17kb long non-coding RNA (lncRNA) which triggers chromosome wide-silencing [150] of the X chromosome from which it is expressed. *XIST* RNA coats the X chromosome in *cis*, followed by recruitment of chromatin remodelling complexes to silence and maintain the inactive status [151, 152].

The earliest step at the onset of XCI is sensing, counting and choosing the X-chromosome to inactivate, thus maintaining a single active X-chromosome per diploid cell. The counting process is presumably *XIST*-independent [151], while choice is influenced by several elements both in *XIST* and *XIC* [153]. An extra element influencing choice in mouse is the X-controlling element (*Xce*) [154], lying in the 3' region to *Xist* [155].

Upregulation of the *XIST* allele from the selected X-chromosome in females occurs upon differentiation. Although not fully understood, change from low levels of biallelic expression to elevated monoallelic *Xist* expression in mouse is apparently under the control of *Tsix*, an antisense-transcribed lncRNA, which acts as a repressor of *Xist* transcription, and is activated in *cis* by *Xite* [156]. These two lncRNAs lie within the *Xic* and are transcribed from the Xa.

New players have been identified in regulation of *Xist/Tsix* expression and X silencing in mouse ES. Among these regulators are positive *Xist* regulators such as *Rnf12,* [157, 158], pluripotency factors that directly repress *Xist* (e.g. *Oct4, Sox2* and *Nanong*), lncRNAs, transcription factors and regulating sequences, which could be either autosomal encoded or X-linked [for a detailed review see 159]. Besides *XIST*, and yet only in a small developmental frame, no other element has been identified to have an essential role in silencing [160-162].

Spread of *XIST* along the X is a gradual process associated to transcription [163], ensuring chromosome-wide silencing and occurring over distances even longer than ~100Mb [164]. XCI signal propagation is enhanced by 'way stations' elements [165] that boost wide and stable X inactivation, probably by recruiting *XIST* or heterchromatin proteins. Long interspersed repeat elements (LINEs) have been proposed as the 'way stations' [166] due to their enrichment originally observed on the human and mouse X [167] and further confirmed on afrotherian and xenarthran X-chromosomes [128]. No obvious accumulation of LINE1 has been reported in marsupials [3], and genomic sequencing of platypus genome rules out enrichment of LINE1 on monotreme sex chromosomes [6], consistent with a *XIST*-independent XCI system in marsupials and an alternative mechanism for balancing expression in monotremes.

Involvement of LINE1s in XCI has been questioned by recent evidence where partial XCI is achieved in autosomal genes after X-to-autosome translocations, where autosomes are not enriched in LINE1s. This has led to the suggestion that LINE1 enrichment could be the nature of the X chromosome, shaped by evolutionary forces like suppression of recombination between X and Y. Besides, additional roles for LINE1s have been hypothesized in escape from X inactivation [159]. Additional elements like GATA repeats, ALU elements and ACG/CGT motifs have been proposed to have a role in XCI [168].

Evolution of the XIST

Even though *XIST* orthologues have been described in eutherian species including the basal placental mammal representative elephant [169], the *XIC* and *XIST* share little homology between human, mouse, cow and vole [170, 171], implying they are poorly conserved in the eutherian lineage. Deletion analysis of *XIST* revealed a region critical for silencing: the A-repeat region, positioned at the proximal end of the *XIST* transcript [172], and it was recently proposed as a positive regulator of *XIST* [173]. In addition, *XIST* exon IV in both human and mouse displays a stem-loop structure [174]. Surprisingly, the A-repeat region and exon IV of *XIST* show high conservation in both sequence and predicted secondary structure in eutherians, including afrotheria and xenarthra [175].

This conservation is suggestive of an *XIST*-dependent X silencing mechanism common to all eutherian mammals. However, the mechanism of regulation and silencing might not be fully conserved. A recent study by Okamoto et al [176] provided evidence that in rabbit and human, XCI starts later than in mouse and *Xist* is originally expressed from both X chromosomes. Furthermore, there is no conservation between human and mouse *TSIX*, the major repressor of *XIST* [170], or *TSIX* mode of repression [177], questioning its role in eutherian *XIST* regulation and the preservation of XCI strategies within the eutherian lineage.

Extensive searches in marsupials have failed to identify an orthologue of the *XIST/TSIX* locus [178]. Bioinformatic and molecular analysis of the region homologous to the eutherian *XIC* show that this region was disturbed in the marsupial and monotreme lineage [175, 178, 179]. Surprisingly the orientation and exonic sequences in four protein-coding genes flanking eutherians *XIST* (from a total of five genes) are conserved in chicken and frogs, potentially representing the ancestral vertebrate arrangement [169, 180, 181]. Although orthologues to these genes were found in opossum and platypus, they map to different regions on the X and chromosome 6, respectively. Examination of the region contained between these flanking genes shows little conservation within eutherians and no obvious homology between eutherians and non-mammals. Genomic sequencing of opossum finally confirmed the absence of *XIST* in marsupials [3], demonstrating its acquirement in eutherians mammals after radiation from marsupials ~148 MYA.

Duret et al [169] proposed a possible origin for *XIST* in the protein-coding gene *LNX3*, which gained a new function after pseudogenization of flanking genes. Comparative genomics reported that opossum maintains a copy of *LNX3* and it is conserved in all vertebrates, with conserved homology between an exon in chicken *LNX3* and *XIST* exon IV [169]. As a functional similarity between *XIST* and *LNX3* seems unlikely [180], an alternative hypothesis establishes *XIST* origin after donation of a transcription-starting site by *LNX3* and integration of a transposable element [182].

XIST and the Suppression of Rearrangements on the X

Conservation of gene content on the X chromosome was first predicted by Ohno, and referred to as "Ohno's Law": the X chromosome is protected against rearrangements that could disrupt the X-inactivation system [80], particularly translocations between the X and autosomes. As mentioned previously, gene content and, for the most part, order is conserved amongst eutherian species but this is not the case for marsupials, where there is extensive rearrangement between the three species for which there is information on gene order [10, 23] (Figure 3). It has been suggested that the suppression of X chromosome rearrangement in the eutherian lineage is due to the *XIST*-mediated silencing mechanism, where the requirement of *XIST* to spread from the *XIC* resulted in selection against rearrangement [3]. The absence of *XIST*, coupled with the highly rearranged nature of genes on the X in marsupials, would support this hypothesis. Additional support is provided by the observation that genes escaping XCI in eutherians are mostly located in the eutherian XAR, which probably has not yet been recruited into the XCI machinery.

Within eutherians, rodents are the exception, where genes from the XAR are intermingled with the XCR (Figure 3). It is interesting to note that the proportion of escaper genes is lower for mouse XAR genes than that observed in elephant and human [141]. A possible explanation is that rearrangements that combined XCR and XAR in mouse facilitated recruitment of XAR genes into the silencing machinery; where inactivation is nearly complete, reflected by little escape from inactivation. Conversely, XAR genes in the rest of the eutherian lineage, where gene order is highly conserved, are still under the gradual process of recruitment. Moreover, the frequency of escaper genes is similar to that observed from X-to-autosome translocations, reflecting recent acquisition of XAR. Interestingly, LINE1 accumulation is lower in regions of the X-chromosome with a higher proportion of escaper genes, particularly on the Xp22, where a long cluster or escaper genes is located [167].

Is there a Marsupial-specific XIC?

The frequent rearrangement of the X in marsupials, together with the absence of *XIST* and the lack of polarity of the level of XCI, was taken as an indication that marsupials lack a marsupial-specific control locus [10, 183]. Astonishingly, recent findings show just the contrary and that there may be such a locus in marsupials. The *RSX* (RNA on the silent X) gene, was identified in opossum, with homologues in Australian marsupials [184]. This gene encodes a ~27 ncRNA that is expressed from the Xi exclusively in females and coats Xi in *cis*, just like *XIST* does. Although *RSX* shares no homology with *XIST*, it bears two highly conserved motifs that could be equivalent to the *XIST* A-repeat and exon IV, as they have the potential to form stem-loops. Expression of *RSX* could not be detected in the female germline, where both X chromosomes remain active, but is expressed in somatic cells where XCI takes place. In addition *RSX* transgenes in mouse ES cells have the potential to coat and silence transgene chromosomes in *cis*. Therefore, *RSX* has been proposed as the marsupial candidate gene regulating XCI [184]. The recent finding of an *XIST*-like ncRNA in marsupials after years of uncertainty, raise the possibility of existence of an homologous locus to *RSX* in monotremes, or even a monotreme-specific locus sharing similar features to those of *RSX* and *XIST*, controlling X-borne gene expression.

Maintaining the Inactive State

In eutherians, once inactivation has been established, the silent status is stably preserved in somatic cells. Maintenance of the X-inactive state is achieved throughout a series of epigenetic modifications. Removal of transcription factors from Xi is one of the immediate events following *XIST* coating, together with displacement of RNA polymerase II from Xi [143, 185]. To achieve transcriptional repression, *XIST* forms a nuclear compartment where non-coding and repetitive sequences are internalized, while coding sequences remain at the periphery [143, 185], allegedly moving inward upon silencing.

Although *XIST* remains permanently associated to Xi, its contribution to transcriptional silencing is limited to early development [162], implying that a silencing partner involved in maintaining XCI still needs to be identified, or that chromatin responsiveness to *XIST* is limited to early developmental stages. *XIST* is involved in XCI initiation and in early maintenance of inactivation through recruitment of Polycomb group proteins [186, 187].

Early variations on the Xi include loss of histone marks associated to active chromatin (H3K4me2, H3K9ac), global H4 hypoacetylation and gain of repressive modifications (H3K9me2, H3K27me3, H4K20me1, H2AK119ub) [reviewed in 152]. Given their early appearance in XCI, these histone modifications could have a role in initiation and maintenance of the inactive state, but their mechanism of action is not fully understood. Once again, comparisons between therian species could help to dissect out the role these modifications play in XCI.

Repressive histone marks are a common feature between marsupials and eutherians. Comparative analysis of the histone modifications profile from opossum, tammar wallaby and elephant suggested a complete enrichment of the repression mark H3K27me3 in elephant and a weaker manifestation in marsupials (30% of nuclei). The H3K27me3 is not exclusively associated with heterochromatin on Xi, indicating that this enrichment is not solely the result of chromatin compaction in marsupials [188].

A striking difference between eutherians and marsupials is the time frame of H3K27me3 accumulation. While this repressive mark is found across the cell cycle in eutherians, its presence in marsupials is transient and begins to accumulate on Xi in early *S* phase, becoming more prominent on late *S* phase and early *G2* phase [188], around the time of Xi replication [123, 189]. This is consistent with previous studies where repressive H3K27me3 mark could not be detected on metaphase chromosomes [190]. This mark is also enriched on opossum Xi at different frequencies in brain and liver tissue [191], suggesting that stability and/or enrichment on Xi could be both tissue-specific or species-specific in marsupials. Both in mouse and marsupials, the Xi is enriched with H3K27me3 usually locates near the nucleolus compartment, possibly to facilitate the recruitment of repressive marks to maintain the heterochromatic state [188]. Notably, *RSX* expression in opossum ovary cells is consistent with enrichment of the H3K27me3 mark, and monoallelic expression of a test X-linked gene (*MSN*) [184]. Marsupial repressive patterns could represent the original epigenetic mechanism for transcriptional silencing that was possibly stabilized upon *XIST* acquisition in the placental lineage.

The conserved chromatin profile within elephant, human and mouse indicates it must have been established ~105 MYA, before placental mammal radiation but after eutherian divergence from marsupials, and has been maintained in all the lineages since then. In addition, active histone modifications (e.g. H3K4me2, H3K9ac, H3K14ac, H3R17me) exhibit differential patterns in Xi compared to Xa in marsupials, as is the case in human, mouse and elephant, suggesting that depletion of marks associated to transcription is a common feature of the Xi [188, 192].

DNA methylation plays a role in epigenetic regulation of gene expression. In human, 5' of CpG islands are methylated on Xi gene promoters, while gene body is hypomethylated [193], probably as a means of stabilization of inactivation. In mouse, methylation status for Xi has been reported to be different to that of Xa in some studies [194], whereas other studies have reported no difference between Xa and Xi methylation patterns [195], making it difficult to conclusively determine the methylation status of mouse Xi. Sequential immunofluorescence on marsupial metaphase chromosomes showed differential methylation where the inactive X is hypomethylated. In platypus, there is no obvious differential methylation in the X-chromosomes, although satellite regions on chromosome 6 and heterochromatic regions show enriched methylation outside sex chromosomes [195]. Methylation of gene promoters occurs at a later stage during XCI and might be responsible for maintaining and stabilizing the inactive X [196]. Searches for DNA methylation on CpG islands from Virginia opossum found that they were hypomethylated on both X chromosomes [197], and bisulfite sequencing detected no methylation difference at the kangaroo *G6PD* locus, or the opossum *G6PD* and *PGK1* loci [40, 198, 199]. However methylation of the maternal X chromosome in kangaroo hybrids was found by *in situ* nick translation [198]. Lack of CpG methylation could explain the less stable nature of marsupial XCI. Further analyses are required to establish the role and significance of DNA methylation in XCI. With the advancement of technology to study CpG methylation status on a genome-wide level, the answer to this long-standing question should be obtained in the near future.

Although individual disruption of XCI marks does not have a great effect on XCI, simultaneous disruption of these marks (i.e. DNA methylation, histone hypoacetylation) together with *XIST* knockout lead to higher reactivation rates of silenced X genes [200], consistent with cooperative regulation of XCI. However, in no case has complete reversal of XCI been achieved, indicating that a major player in XCI regulation might still remain unidentified. For instance, various authors have proposed the existence of a molecule replacing *XIST* in later developmental stages. Perhaps, further epigenetic variations on the Xi, acting at different stages and in different cell-types are yet to be identified.

In monotremes, epigenetic patterns are not similar to that of therians. Rens et al [195] observed no difference in patterns for active or repressive marks between the two copies of X chromosomes in females, and reported absence of differential histone acetylation patterns between platypus autosomes and sex chromosomes. This indicates that global X upregulation does not occur in platypus; however, as discussed earlier in this chapter, dosage compensation studies suggest that the X chromosome is upregulated in males, or in both sexes, followed by silencing of the female Xs [104]. This discrepancy can be explained by a gene-by-gene upregulation in both sexes and further gene-by-gene inactivation in females as previously proposed. Alternatively, monotremes could have different epigenetic marks to that of therians, which have not yet been identified.

Hypotheses for the Evolution of XCI

Since the discovery of XCI in therian mammals, the primary question that has been posed is whether XCI in marsupials and eutherians shared a common ancestry or arose independently in each lineage. In this chapter, we have highlighted the conservation of gene content of therian X chromosomes, which may suggest a common origin of the XCI mechanism, but we have also noted the striking differences in XCI features between the two lineages (Table 1). As a result, the precise route of XCI evolution is unknown and several evolutionary scenarios have been proposed.

The evolution of this remarkable epigenetic phenomenon has been inextricably linked to the degradation of the Y chromosome. Comparative analysis of the genes on marsupial and eutherian Y chromosomes suggests independent degradation of the Y chromosome [201], resulting in independent genesis of XCI systems in the marsupial and eutherian lineages [183]. Analysis of gene retrotransposition from the X to autosomes shows that most retrotransposition events occurred independently in the marsupial and eutherian lineages, implying that the majority of differentiation between the X and Y chromosomes occurred after marsupial/eutherian divergence [41, 42].

In addition, the key gene responsible for the suppression of recombination between the proto-X and Y chromosomes is the testis determining factor, which in therian mammals is *SRY* and is derived from the X-borne gene *SOX3*. Gribnau and Grootegoed [202] suggested that the XCI system, at least in eutherian mammals, is likely to have arisen in the region encompassing *SOX3*, as high doses of the SOX3 protein are able to trigger the testis differentiation pathway [203], making *SOX3* a dosage-sensitive gene. The *LNX3* gene from which *XIST* adopted a transcription start site, along with other key genes in the eutherian XCI mechanism, are located in close proximity to *SOX3* on the proto-X, supporting this idea. In contrast, *SOX3* in marsupials does not share the same role as the eutherian *SOX3* gene and it is not expressed in developing testes as it is in eutherians [204], suggesting that *SOX3* in marsupials may not be dosage-sensitive and therefore unlikely to be the location at which X chromosome inactivation arose. This would suggest an independent origin of XCI in marsupials and eutherians. Furthermore, the marsupial-specific lnc-

RNA *RSX* is located in a different region of the proto-X chromosome, adjacent to *HPRT1* and *PHF6X*.

Table 1. Features of X chromosome inactivation in eutherians, marsupials and monotremes

	Eutherians	Marsupials	Monotremes
Controlling locus	*XIST*	*RSX*	?
LINE1 Accumulation	Yes	No	No
Barr body formation	Yes	CD	No
Asyncrhonous Replication	Yes	Yes	Yes (specific regions)
Chromosome-wide Inactivation	Yes	Yes	? (at least regional inactivation)
Random Inactivation	Somatic tissues	No	Yes
Imprinted Inactivation	Extraembryonic tissues of mouse, cattle	Yes	No
Inactivation Status	Essentially complete for XCR Incomplete for XAR	Incomplete	Incomplete
Depletion of active histone marks	Yes	Yes	No
Repressive histone marks	Yes	Yes	No
CpG methylation	Yes	CD	No (cytogenetically determined)

CD Conflicting data.
? Unknown.

Alternatively, it is possible that XCI evolved from a mechanism present in the common ancestor of therian mammals, which has gained added levels of complexity in the eutherian lineage to manifest as the highly stable and more complete silencing system we observe today. Upon discovery of paternal X inactivation in marsupials, Cooper [205] proposed that random XCI observed in eutherians was derived from an ancestral imprinted form of XCI, which has been retained in marsupials.

Finding imprinted XCI in the extraembryonic tissues of rodents [206-208] and cattle [209] supported this hypothesis, yet imprinted XCI is not universal in the extraembryonic tissues of eutherians. Random XCI has been reported in human placentae [210] and reciprocal crosses of hybrid placenta tissue of horse and donkey [211]. The less stable nature of inactivation and lack of involvement of DNA methylation [212, 213] shared between marsupial and eutherian imprinted XCI would support a common ancestry except for one important difference, which is the involvement of *Xist* in imprinted XCI in mice [214, 215], although it is perhaps less dependent on *Xist* than random XCI [216]. Alternative epigenetic mechanisms, like Polycomb group proteins could be more significant for XCI in extraembryonic tissues [217, 218]. This could explain differential stability and epigenetic modifications according to developmental stage and cell lineage, where extraembryonic tissues could cope with a less tight repression system as they would be discarded after birth, while in embryonic lineages, longer-term silencing is required as these tissues develop into the soma. Interestingly, the placenta is the only tissue where XCI reversal has been achieved *in situ* [219].

The paternal X in mouse extraembryonic tissues does not share the same histone modification signature as marsupials, but is similar to that of random XCI [188]. Furthermore, recent comparative studies propose a later origin of imprinted XCI in extraembryonic tissues of mice [220]. Thus, strategies for imprinted XCI must have evolved independently in marsupials and eutherian extraembryonic tissues.

MSCI has been suggested as the precursor of somatic imprinted X inactivation in marsupials [39, 40, 124, 221]. The marsupial X and Y chromosomes are silenced during male meiosis at pachytene stage and are stably maintained along spermiogenesis [222]. Thus, the zygote could receive an already inactive X from the sperm. Reactivation of X-linked genes in spermatids in opossum, and to a lesser extent in mouse [191], and the difficulties of transmitting epigenetic marks through sperm compromise this hypothesis.

Another possibility for the origin of XCI is that it arose from an ancient mechanism to regulate transcription that has been exapted into an independently evolved mechanism to equalise the expression of dosage-sensitive genes. In monotremes, this presents as a stochastic form of expression in females, where silencing one allele in approximately 50% of nuclei provides a sufficient level of male to female compensation [140]. In marsupials, imprinted XCI appears, at least in some cell types, to be incomplete and is due to stochastic expression from the inactive X [183]. Despite the more complete inactivation of genes in the eutherian XCR, those from the XAR are more prone to a stochastic form of expression. This type of expression may be indicative of the ancestral mechanism as this represents a recent addition to the X, which is yet to be recruited into the more stable and complete form of inactivation apparent for the XCR. The recruitment of extra layers of control, such as histone modifications and 5' CpG methylation, contribute to this more complex yet stable form of XCI.

This stochastic hypothesis is not limited to the evolution of XCI but may be a more general mechanism for regulating transcription from which genomic imprinting [223] or, even the now more widely observed random monoallelic expression of some genes [224], has evolved, with layers of epigenetic complexity added depending on selective pressures.

Conclusion

Sequencing of genomes from distantly related mammals has had a huge impact on our understanding of the evolution of mammalian sex chromosomes and the mechanisms that have evolved to compensate for differences in transcriptional output between the X and autosomes, as well as between males and females. For instance, the age of the therian sex chromosomes is much younger than previously supposed and this has in turn influenced the proposed models for the evolution of XCI. It was once thought that efficient dosage compensation was critical for life, but it has become more apparent that only a subset of genes on the X require strict compensation and most genes are tolerant of dosage differences. While we now have a good grasp on the evolution of mammalian sex chromosomes, the evolution of compensation mechanisms, whether to equalize transcriptional output between the X chromosome and autosomes or between males and females, is obviously very complex. A comparative analysis of the intricacies of these mechanisms will enable the pieces of the evolutionary puzzle surrounding them to be pieced together.

Acknowledgments

C.L.R.D. is supported by a CONACyT scholarship from the Mexican Government and an Australian Research Council Discovery grant awarded to P. Waters, J. Deakin and J. Graves. J.E.D is supported by an Australian Research Council Future Fellowship.

References

[1] Bellott, D.W., et al., *Convergent evolution of chicken Z and human X chromosomes by expansion and gene acquisition.* Nature, 2010. 466(7306): p. 612-6.

[2] Bininda-Emonds, O.R., et al., *The delayed rise of present-day mammals.* Nature, 2007. 446(7135): p. 507-12.

[3] Mikkelsen, T.S., et al., *Genome of the marsupial Monodelphis domestica reveals innovation in non-coding sequences.* Nature, 2007. 447(7141): p. 167-77.

[4] Renfree, M.B., et al., *Genome sequence of an Australian kangaroo, Macropus eugenii, provides insight into the evolution of mammalian reproduction and development.* Genome Biol, 2011. 12(8): p. R81.

[5] Flannery, T.F. and C.P. Groves, *A revision of the genus Zaglossus (Monotremata, Tachyglossidae) with description of new species and subspecies.* Mammalia, 1998. 62: p. 367-396.

[6] Warren, W.C., et al., *Genome analysis of the platypus reveals unique signatures of evolution.* Nature, 2008. 453(7192): p. 175-83.

[7] Muller, H., *A gene for the fourth chromosome of Drosophila.* Journal of Experimental Zoology, 1914. 17(3):p. 325-336.

[8] Charlesworth, B. and D. Charlesworth, *The degeneration of Y chromosomes.* Philosophical transactions of the Royal Society of London. Series B, Biological Sciences, 2000. 355(1403): p. 1563-72.

[9] Wilson, M.A. and K.D. Makova, *Evolution and survival on eutherian sex chromosomes.* PLoS Genet, 2009. 5(7).

[10] Deakin, J.E., et al., *Physical map of two tammar wallaby chromosomes: a strategy for mapping in non-model mammals.* Chromosome Res, 2008. 16(8): p. 1159-75.

[11] Spencer, J.A., J.M. Watson, and J.A. Graves, *The X chromosome of marsupials shares a highly conserved region with eutherians.* Genomics, 1991. 9(4): p. 598-604.

[12] Glas, R., et al., *Cross-species chromosome painting between human and marsupial directly demonstrates the ancient region of the mammalian X.* Mammalian genome : official journal of the International Mammalian Genome Society, 1999. 10(11): p. 1115-6.

[13] Graves, J.A., *The evolution of mammalian sex chromosomes and the origin of sex determining genes.* Philos Trans R Soc Lond B Biol Sci, 1995. 350(1333): p. 305-11; discussion 311-2.

[14] Spencer, J.A., et al., *Genes on the short arm of the human X chromosome are not shared with the marsupial X.* Genomics, 1991. 11(2): p. 339-45.

[15] Wilcox, S.A., et al., *Comparative mapping identifies the fusion point of an ancient mammalian X-autosomal rearrangement.* Genomics, 1996. 35(1): p. 66-70.

[16] Ross, M.T., et al., *The DNA sequence of the human X chromosome.* Nature, 2005. 434(7031): p. 325-37.

[17] Rodriguez Delgado, C.L., et al., *Physical mapping of the elephant X chromosome: conservation of gene order over 105 million years.* Chromosome Research, 2009. 17(7): p. 917-26.

[18] Murphy, W.J., et al., *Extensive conservation of sex chromosome organization between cat and human revealed by parallel radiation hybrid mapping.* Genome Research, 1999. 9(12): p. 1223-30.

[19] Band, M.R., et al., *An ordered comparative map of the cattle and human genomes.* Genome Research, 2000. 10(9): p. 1359-68.

[20] Swinburne, J.E., et al., *Single linkage group per chromosome genetic linkage map for the horse, based on two three-generation, full-sibling, crossbred horse reference families.* Genomics, 2006. 87(1): p. 1-29.

[21] Gibbs, R.A., et al., *Genome sequence of the Brown Norway rat yields insights into mammalian evolution.* Nature, 2004. 428(6982): p. 493-521.

[22] Vilella, A.J., et al., *EnsemblCompara GeneTrees: Complete, duplication-aware phylogenetic trees in vertebrates.* Genome Research, 2009. 19(2): p. 327-35.

[23] Deakin, J.E., et al., *Genomic restructuring in the Tasmanian devil facial tumour: chromosome painting and gene mapping provide clues to evolution of a transmissible tumour.* PLoS Genet, 2012. 8(2): p. e1002483.

[24] Mueller, J.L., et al., *The mouse X chromosome is enriched for multicopy testis genes showing postmeiotic expression.* Nature Genetics, 2008. 40(6): p. 794-9.

[25] Warburton, P.E., et al., *Inverted repeat structure of the human genome: the X-chromosome contains a preponderance of large, highly homologous inverted repeats that contain testes genes.* Genome Research, 2004. 14(10A): p. 1861-9.

[26] Delbridge, M.L. and J.A. Graves, *Origin and evolution of spermatogenesis genes on the human sex chromosomes.* Society of Reproduction and Fertility supplement, 2007. 65: p. 1-17.

[27] Saifi, G.M. and H.S. Chandra, *An apparent excess of sex- and repdroduction- related genes on the human X chromosome.* Philosophical transactions of the Royal Society of London. Series B, Biological Sciences, 1999. 266: p. 203-209.

[28] Wang, P.J., et al., *An abundance of X-linked genes expressed in spermatogonia.* Nature Genetics, 2001. 27(4): p. 422-6.

[29] Khil, P.P., et al., *The mouse X chromosome is enriched for sex-biased genes not subject to selection by meiotic sex chromosome inactivation.* Nature Genetics, 2004. 36(6): p. 642-6.

[30] Koslowski, M., et al., *The human X chromosome is enriched for germline genes expressed in premeiotic germ cells of both sexes.* Human Molecular Genetics, 2006. 15(15): p. 2392-9.

[31] Wilda, M., et al., *Do the constraints of human speciation cause expression of the same set of genes in brain, testis, and placenta?* Cytogenetics and Cell Genetics, 2000. 91(1-4): p. 300-2.

[32] Graves, J.A., J. Gecz, and H. Hameister, *Evolution of the human X--a smart and sexy chromosome that controls speciation and development.* Cytogenetic and Genome Research, 2002. 99(1-4): p. 141-5.

[33] Delbridge, M.L., et al., *Origin and evolution of candidate mental retardation genes on the human X chromosome (MRX).* BMC Genomics, 2008. 9: p. 65.

[34] Turner, R.M., et al., *An X-linked gene encodes a major human sperm fibrous sheath protein, hAKAP82. Genomic organization, protein kinase A-RII binding, and distribution of the precursor in the sperm tail.* The Journal of Biological Chemistry, 1998. 273(48): p. 32135-41.

[35] Hu, Y., et al., *A-kinase anchoring protein 4 has a conserved role in mammalian spermatogenesis.* Reproduction, 2009. 137(4): p. 645-53.

[36] Hu, Y., et al., *Kallmann syndrome 1 gene is expressed in the marsupial gonad.* Biology of Reproduction, 2011. 84(3): p. 595-603.

[37] Hu, Y., et al., *Differential roles of TGIF family genes in mammalian reproduction.* BMC Developmental Biology, 2011. 11: p. 58.
[38] Kohn, M., et al., *Recruitment of old genes to new functions: evidences obtained by comparing the orthologues of human XLMR genes in mouse and chicken.* Cytogenetic and Genome Research, 2007. 116(3): p. 173-80.
[39] Namekawa, S.H., et al., *Sex chromosome silencing in the marsupial male germ line.* Proceedings of the National Academy of Sciences of the United States of America, 2007. 104(23): p. 9730-5.
[40] Hornecker, J.L., et al., *Meiotic sex chromosome inactivation in the marsupial Monodelphis domestica.* Genesis, 2007. 45(11): p. 696-708.
[41] McLysaght, A., *Evolutionary steps of sex chromosomes are reflected in retrogenes.* Trends in Genetics : TIG, 2008. 24(10): p. 478-81.
[42] Potrzebowski, L., et al., *Chromosomal gene movements reflect the recent origin and biology of therian sex chromosomes.* PLoS Biology, 2008. 6(4): p. e80.
[43] Emerson, J.J., et al., *Extensive gene traffic on the mammalian X chromosome.* Science, 2004. 303(5657): p. 537-40.
[44] Rens, W., et al., *Resolution and evolution of the duck-billed platypus karyotype with an X1Y1X2Y2X3Y3X4Y4X5Y5 male sex chromosome constitution.* Proc Natl Acad Sci U S A, 2004. 101(46): p. 16257-61.
[45] Grutzner, F., et al., *In the platypus a meiotic chain of ten sex chromosomes shares genes with the bird Z and mammal X chromosomes.* Nature, 2004. 432(7019): p. 913-7.
[46] Rens, W., et al., *The multiple sex chromosomes of platypus and echidna are not completely identical and several share homology with the avian Z.* Genome Biol, 2007. 8(11): p. R243.
[47] Gruetzner, F., et al., *How did the platypus get its sex chromosome chain? A comparison of meiotic multiples and sex chromosomes in plants and animals.* Chromosoma, 2006. 115(2): p. 75-88.
[48] Rens, W., et al., *Resolution and evolution of the duck-billed platypus karyotype with an X1Y1X2Y2X3Y3X4Y4X5Y5 male sex chromosome constitution.* Proceedings of the National Academy of Sciences of the United States of America, 2004. 101(46): p. 16257-61.
[49] Rens, W., et al., *The multiple sex chromosomes of platypus and echidna are not completely identical and several share homology with the avian Z.* Genome Biology, 2007. 8(11): p. R243.
[50] Ashley, T., *Chromosome chains and platypus sex: kinky connections.* Bioessays, 2005. 27(7): p. 681-4.

[51] Wrigley, J.M. and J.A. Graves, *Sex chromosome homology and incomplete, tissue-specific X-inactivation suggest that monotremes represent an intermediate stage of mammalian sex chromosome evolution.* J Hered, 1988. 79(2): p. 115-8.
[52] Veyrunes, F., et al., *Bird-like sex chromosomes of platypus imply recent origin of mammal sex chromosomes.* Genome Res, 2008. 18(6): p. 965-73.
[53] Raudsepp, T. and B.P. Chowdhary, *The horse pseudoautosomal region (PAR): characterization and comparison with the human, chimp and mouse PARs.* Cytogenetic and Genome Research, 2008. 121(2): p. 102-9.
[54] Van Laere, A.S., W. Coppieters, and M. Georges, *Characterization of the bovine pseudoautosomal boundary: Documenting the evolutionary history of mammalian sex chromosomes.* Genome Research, 2008. 18(12): p. 1884-95.
[55] Ratomponirina, C., et al., *Synaptonemal complexes in Gerbillidae: probable role of intercalated heterochromatin in gonosome-autosome translocations.* Cytogenetics and Cell Genetics, 1986. 43(3-4): p. 161-7.
[56] Ratomponirina, C., et al., *Synaptonemal complex study in some species of Gerbillidae without heterochromatin interposition.* Cytogenetics and Cell Genetics, 1989. 52(1-2): p. 23-7.
[57] Ashley, T., M. Jaarola, and K. Fredga, *Absence of synapsis during pachynema of the normal sized sex chromosomes of Microtus arvalis.* Hereditas, 1989. 111(3): p. 295-304.
[58] Carnero, A., et al., *Achiasmatic sex chromosomes in Pitymys duodecimcostatus: mechanisms of association and segregation.* Cytogenetics and Cell Genetics, 1991. 56(2): p. 78-81.
[59] Jimenez, R., et al., *Achiasmatic giant sex chromosomes in the vole Microtus cabrerae (Rodentia, Microtidae).* Cytogenetics and Cell Genetics, 1991. 57(1): p. 56-8.
[60] Wolf, K.W., K. Baumgart, and H. Winking, *Meiotic association and segregation of the achiasmatic giant sex chromosomes in the male field vole (Microtus agrestis).* Chromosoma, 1988. 97(2): p. 124-33.
[61] Graves, J.A., *Mammals that break the rules: genetics of marsupials and monotremes.* Annual Review of Genetics, 1996. 30: p. 233-60.
[62] Graves, J.A., M.J. Wakefield, and R. Toder, *The origin and evolution of the pseudoautosomal regions of human sex chromosomes.* Human Molecular Genetics, 1998. 7(13): p. 1991-6.

[63] Page, J., et al., *The pairing of X and Y chromosomes during meiotic prophase in the marsupial species Thylamys elegans is maintained by a dense plate developed from their axial elements.* Journal of Cell Science, 2003. 116(Pt 3): p. 551-60.
[64] Fernandez-Donoso, R., S. Berrios, and J. Pincheira, *Position of the nucleolus within the nuclei of pachytene spermatocytes of Dromiciops australis and Marmosa elegans (Didelphoidea-Marsupialia).* Experientia, 1979. 35(8): p. 1021-3.
[65] Tres, L.L., *XY chromosomal bivalent: nucleolar attraction.* Molecular Reproduction and Development, 2005. 72(1): p. 1-6.
[66] Berrios, S. and R. Fernandez-Donoso, *Nuclear architecture of human pachytene spermatocytes: quantitative analysis of associations between nucleolar and XY bivalents.* Human Genetics, 1990. 86(2): p. 103-16.
[67] Liu, J., *Control of protein synthesis and mRNA degradation by microRNAs.* Current Opinion in Cell Biology, 2008. 20(2): p. 214-21.
[68] Heimberg, A.M., et al., *MicroRNAs and the advent of vertebrate morphological complexity.* Proceedings of the National Academy of Sciences of the United States of America, 2008. 105(8): p. 2946-50.
[69] Guo, X., et al., *Rapid evolution of mammalian X-linked testis microRNAs.* BMC Genomics, 2009. 10: p. 97.
[70] Zhang, R., et al., *Rapid evolution of an X-linked microRNA cluster in primates.* Genome Research, 2007. 17(5): p. 612-7.
[71] Yu, Z., T. Raabe, and N.B. Hecht, *MicroRNA Mirn122a reduces expression of the posttranscriptionally regulated germ cell transition protein 2 (Tnp2) messenger RNA (mRNA) by mRNA cleavage.* Biology of Reproduction, 2005. 73(3): p. 427-33.
[72] Ro, S., et al., *Cloning and expression profiling of testis-expressed microRNAs.* Developmental Biology, 2007. 311(2): p. 592-602.
[73] Murchison, E.P., et al., *Conservation of small RNA pathways in platypus.* Genome Research, 2008. 18(6): p. 995-1004.
[74] Devor, E.J. and P.B. Samollow, *In vitro and in silico annotation of conserved and nonconserved microRNAs in the genome of the marsupial Monodelphis domestica.* The Journal of Heredity, 2008. 99(1): p. 66-72.
[75] Devor, E.J., et al., *An X chromosome microRNA cluster in the marsupial species Monodelphis domestica.* The Journal of Heredity, 2011. 102(5): p. 577-83.
[76] Li, J., et al., *Evolution of an X-linked primate-specific micro RNA cluster.* Molecular Biology and Evolution, 2010. 27(3): p. 671-83.

[77] Hughes, J.F., et al., *Chimpanzee and human Y chromosomes are remarkably divergent in structure and gene content.* Nature, 2010. 463(7280): p. 536-9.

[78] Skaletsky, H., et al., *The male-specific region of the human Y chromosome is a mosaic of discrete sequence classes.* Nature, 2003. 423(6942): p. 825-37.

[79] Toder, R., M.J. Wakefield, and J.A. Graves, *The minimal mammalian Y chromosome - the marsupial Y as a model system.* Cytogenetics and Cell Genetics, 2000. 91(1-4): p. 285-92.

[80] Ohno, S., *Sex chromosomes and sex-linked genes.(Monographs on endocrinology, Vol. 1.).* Sex chromosomes and sex-linked genes.(Monographs on endocrinology, Vol. 1.), 1967.

[81] Payer, B. and J.T. Lee, *X chromosome dosage compensation: how mammals keep the balance.* Annual Review of Genetics, 2008. 42: p. 733-72.

[82] Straub, T. and P. Becker, *Dosage compensation: the beginning and end of generalization.* Nature Reviews. Genetics, 2007. 8(1): p. 47-57.

[83] Heard, E. and C. Disteche, *Dosage compensation in mammals: fine-tuning the expression of the X chromosome.* Genes & Development, 2006. 20(14): p. 1848-67.

[84] Nguyen, D.K. and C.M. Disteche, *Dosage compensation of the active X chromosome in mammals.* Nature genetics, 2006. 38(1): p. 47-53.

[85] Lucchesi, J., *Dosage compensation in Drosophila.* Annual review of genetics, 1973. 7: p. 225-37.

[86] Ercan, S., et al., *X chromosome repression by localization of the C. elegans dosage compensation machinery to sites of transcription initiation.* Nature Genetics, 2007. 39(3): p. 403-8.

[87] Adler, D., et al., *Evidence of evolutionary up-regulation of the single active X chromosome in mammals based on Clc4 expression levels in Mus spretus and Mus musculus.* Proceedings of the National Academy of Sciences of the United States of America, 1997. 94(17): p. 9244-48.

[88] Lin, H., et al., *Dosage compensation in the mouse balances up-regulation and silencing of X-linked genes.* PLoS Biology, 2007. 5(12): p. e326.

[89] Khaitovich, P., et al., *Evolution of primate gene expression.* Nature Reviews. Genetics, 2006. 7(9): p. 693-702.

[90] Castagné, R.l., et al., *The choice of the filtering method in microarrays affects the inference regarding dosage compensation of the active X-chromosome.* PLoS One, 2011. 6(9): e23956.

[91] Xiong, Y., et al., *RNA sequencing shows no dosage compensation of the active X-chromosome.* Nat Genet, 2010. 42(12): p. 1043-7.
[92] Deng, X., et al., *Evidence for compensatory upregulation of expressed X-linked genes in mammals, Caenorhabditis elegans and Drosophila melanogaster.* Nat Genet, 2011. 43(12): p. 1179-85.
[93] Yildirim, E., et al., *X-chromosome hyperactivation in mammals via nonlinear relationships between chromatin states and transcription.* Nature Structural & Molecular Biology, 2012. 19(1): p. 56-61.
[94] Phatnani, H.P. and A.L. Greenleaf, *Phosphorylation and functions of the RNA polymerase II CTD.* Genes & Development, 2006. 20(21): p. 2922-36.
[95] Bernstein, B., et al., *Genomic maps and comparative analysis of histone modifications in human and mouse.* Cell, 2005. 120(2): p. 169-81.
[96] Schneider, R., et al., *Histone H3 lysine 4 methylation patterns in higher eukaryotic genes.* Nature Cell Biology, 2004. 6(1): p. 73-77.
[97] He, X., et al., *He et al. reply.* Nat Genet, 2011. 43(12): p. 1171-1172.
[98] Kharchenko, P., R. Xi, and P. Park, *Evidence for dosage compensation between the X chromosome and autosomes in mammals.* Nature genetics, 2011. 43(12): p. 1167-69.
[99] Lin, H., et al., *Relative overexpression of X-linked genes in mouse embryonic stem cells is consistent with Ohno's hypothesis.* Nature genetics, 2011. 43(12): p. 1169-70.
[100] Mank, J.E., D.J. Hosken, and N. Wedell, *Some inconvenient truths about sex chromosome dosage compensation and the potential role of sexual conflict.* Evolution, 2011. 65(8): p. 2133-44.
[101] Pessia, E., et al., *Mammalian X chromosome inactivation evolved as a dosage-compensation mechanism for dosage-sensitive genes on the X chromosome.* Proc Natl Acad Sci U S A, 2012. 109(14): p. 5346-51.
[102] Lin, F., et al., *Expression reduction in mammalian X chromosome evolution refutes Ohno's hypothesis of dosage compensation.* Proceedings of the National Academy of Sciences of the United States of America, 2012. 109(29): p. 11752-7.
[103] Julien, P., et al., *Mechanisms and evolutionary patterns of Mammalian and avian dosage compensation.* PLoS Biology, 2012. 10(5): p. e1001328.
[104] Al Nadaf, S., et al., *Activity map of the tammar X chromosome shows that marsupial X inactivation is incomplete and escape is stochastic.* Genome Biology, 2010. 11(12): p. R122.

[105] Deakin, J.E., et al., *The status of dosage compensation in the multiple X chromosomes of the platypus.* PLoS Genetics, 2008. 4(7): p. e1000140.
[106] Itoh, Y., et al., *Dosage compensation is less effective in birds than in mammals.* Journal of biology, 2007. 6(1): p. 2.
[107] Ellegren, H., et al., *Faced with inequality: chicken do not have a general dosage compensation of sex-linked genes.* BMC biology, 2007. 5: p. 40.
[108] Deakin, J.E., et al., *Unravelling the evolutionary origins of X chromosome inactivation in mammals: insights from marsupials and monotremes.* Chromosome Research, 2009. 17(5): p. 671-85.
[109] Charlesworth, B., *The evolution of chromosomal sex determination and dosage compensation.* Current Biology : CB, 1996. 6(2): p. 149-62.
[110] Lahn, B.T., N.M. Pearson, and K. Jegalian, *The human Y chromosome, in the light of evolution.* Nature Reviews. Genetics, 2001. 2(3): p. 207-16.
[111] Payer, B. and J.T. Lee, *X chromosome dosage compensation: how mammals keep the balance.* Annual Review of Genetics, 2008. 42: p. 733-72.
[112] Makino, T. and A. McLysaght, *Ohnologs in the human genome are dosage balanced and frequently associated with disease.* Proceedings of the National Academy of Sciences of the United States of America, 2010. 107(20): p. 9270-4.
[113] Graves, J.A. and C.M. Disteche, *Does gene dosage really matter?* Journal of Biology, 2007. 6(1): p. 1.
[114] Lucchesi, J.C., W.G. Kelly, and B. Panning, *Chromatin remodeling in dosage compensation.* Annual Review of Genetics, 2005. 39: p. 615-51.
[115] Lyon, M.F., *Gene action in the X-chromosome of the mouse (Mus musculus L.).* Nature, 1961. 190: p. 372-3.
[116] Gendrel, A.V. and E. Heard, *Fifty years of X-inactivation research.* Development, 2011. 138(23): p. 5049-55.
[117] Beutler, E., M. Yeh, and V.F. Fairbanks, *The normal human female as a mosaic of X-chromosome activity: studies using the gene for C-6-PD-deficiency as a marker.* Proceedings of the National Academy of Sciences of the United States of America, 1962. 48: p. 9-16.
[118] Davidson, R.G., H.M. Nitowsky, and B. Childs, *Demonstration of Two Populations of Cells in the Human Female Heterozygous for Glucose-6-Phosphate Dehydrogenase Variants.* Proc Natl Acad Sci U S A, 1963. 50: p. 481-5.
[119] Barr, M.L. and D.H. Carr, *Correlations between sex chromatin and sex chromosomes.* Acta Cytol, 1962. 6: p. 34-45.

[120] Taylor, J.H., *Asynchronous duplication of chromosomes in cultured cells of Chinese hamster.* J Biophys Biochem Cytol, 1960. 7: p. 455-64.
[121] Graves, J.A., *DNA synthesis in chromosomes of cultured leucocytes from two marsupial species.* Exp Cell Res, 1967. 46(1): p. 37-57.
[122] Sharman, G.B., *Late DNA replication in the paternally derived X chromosome of female kangaroos.* Nature, 1971. 230(5291): p. 231-2.
[123] Cooper, D.W., et al., *Phosphoglycerate kinase polymorphism in kangaroos provides further evidence for paternal X inactivation.* Nature: New biology, 1971. 230(13): p. 155-7.
[124] Richardson, B.J., A.B. Czuppon, and G.B. Sharman, *Inheritance of glucose-6-phosphate dehydrogenase variation in kangaroos.* Nature: New biology, 1971. 230(13): p. 154-5.
[125] Cooper, D.W., P.G. Johnston, and J.A.M. Graves, *X-inactivation in marsupials and monotremes.* Seminars in cell & developmental biology, 1993. 4: p. 117-128.
[126] Cooper, D.W., et al., *X-Chromosome Inactivation in Marsupials.* Aust J Zool, 1990. 37(2-4): p. 411-417.
[127] Waters, P.D., et al., *Sex chromosomes of basal placental mammals.* Chromosoma, 2007. 116(6): p. 511-8.
[128] Johnston, P.G. and E.S. Robinson, *X chromosome inactivation in female embryos of a marsupial mouse (Antechinus stuartii).* Chromosoma, 1987. 95(6): p. 419-23.
[129] McKay, L.M., J.M. Wrigley, and J.A. Graves, *Evolution of mammalian X-chromosome inactivation: sex chromatin in monotremes and marsupials.* Australian Journal of Biological Sciences, 1987. 40(4): p. 397-404.
[130] Ho, K.K.K., et al., *Replication asynchrony and differential condensation of X chromosomes in female platypus (Ornithorhynchus anatinus).* Reproduction, Fertility and Development, 2009. 21: p. 952-963.
[131] Murtagh, C.E., *A unique cytogenetic system in monotremes.* Chromosoma, 1977. 65: p. 37-57.
[132] Carrel, L. and H.F. Willard, *X-inactivation profile reveals extensive variability in X-linked gene expression in females.* Nature, 2005. 434(7031): p. 400-4.
[133] Johnston, C.M., et al., *Large-scale population study of human cell lines indicates that dosage compensation is virtually complete.* PLoS Genetics, 2008. 4(1): p. e9.
[134] VandeBerg, J.L., et al., *Studies on metatherian sex chromosomes. IV. X linkage of PGK-A with paternal X inactivation confirmed in erythrocytes*

of grey kangaroos by pedigree analysis. Australian Journal of Biological Sciences, 1977. 30(1-2): p. 115-25.

[135] Vandeberg, J.L., D.W. Cooper, and G.B. Sharman, *Phosphoglycerate kinase A polymorphism in the wallaby Macropus parryi: activity of both X chromosomes in muscle.* Nature (London) New Biol, 1973. 243: p. 47-8.

[136] Cooper, D.W., et al., *Studies on metatherian sex chromosomes VI. A third state of an X-linked gene: partial activity for the paternally derived Pgk-A allele in cultured fibroblasts of Macropus giganteus and M. parryi.* Aust J Biol Sci, 1977. 30: p. 431-443.

[137] Johnston, P.G., et al., *Studies on metatherian sex chromosomes VII. Glucose-6-phosphate dehydrogenase expression in tissues and cultured fibroblasts of kangaroos.* Aust J Biol Sci, 1978. 31: p. 415-424.

[138] Livernois, A.M., et al., *Independent evolution of transcriptional inactivation on sex chromosomes in birds on sex chromosomes in birds and mammals.* submitted.

[139] Deakin, J.E., et al., *The status of dosage compensation in the multiple X chromosomes of the platypus.* PLoS Genet, 2008. 4(7): p. e1000140.

[140] Al Nadaf, S., et al., *A cross-species comparison of escape from X inactivation in Eutheria: implications for evolution of X chromosome inactivation.* Chromosoma, 2012. 121(1): p. 71-8.

[141] Yang, F., et al., *Global survey of escape from X inactivation by RNA-sequencing in mouse.* Genome Res, 2010. 20(5): p. 614-22.

[142] Chaumeil, J., et al., *A novel role for Xist RNA in the formation of a repressive nuclear compartment into which genes are recruited when silenced.* Genes & development, 2006. 20(16): p. 2223-37.

[143] Graves, J.A., C.M. Disteche, and R. Toder, *Gene dosage in the evolution and function of mammalian sex chromosomes.* Cytogenetics and cell genetics, 1998. 80(1-4): p. 94-103.

[144] Kuroda, Y., et al., *Absence of Z-chromosome inactivation for five genes in male chickens.* Chromosome Research, 2001. 9(6): p. 457-68.

[145] Kuroiwa, A., et al., *Biallelic expression of Z-linked genes in male chickens.* Cytogenetic and Genome Research, 2002. 99(1-4): p. 310-4.

[146] Morey, C. and P. Avner, *The demoiselle of X-inactivation: 50 years old and as trendy and mesmerising as ever.* PLoS Genet, 2011. 7(7): p. e1002212.

[147] Brown, C.J., et al., *Localization of the X inactivation centre on the human X chromosome in Xq13.* Nature, 1991. 349(6304): p. 82-4.

[148] Lee, J.T., N. Lu, and Y. Han, *Genetic analysis of the mouse X inactivation center defines an 80-kb multifunction domain.* Proc Natl Acad Sci U S A, 1999. 96(7): p. 3836-41.
[149] Borsani, G., et al., *Characterization of a murine gene expressed from the inactive X chromosome.* Nature, 1991. 351(6324): p. 325-9.
[150] Avner, P. and E. Heard, *X-chromosome inactivation: counting, choice and initiation.* Nature reviews. Genetics, 2001. 2(1): p. 59-67.
[151] Heard, E., *Delving into the diversity of facultative heterochromatin: the epigenetics of the inactive X chromosome.* Current Opinion in Genetics & Development, 2005. 15(5): p. 482-9.
[152] Marahrens, Y., J. Loring, and R. Jaenisch, *Role of the Xist gene in X chromosome choosing.* Cell, 1998. 92(5): p. 657-64.
[153] Cattanach, B.M. and C.E. Williams, *Evidence of non-random X chromosome activity in the mouse.* Genet Res, 1972. 19(3): p. 229-40.
[154] Simmler, M.C., et al., *Mapping the murine Xce locus with (CA)n repeats.* Mamm Genome, 1993. 4(9): p. 523-30.
[155] Lee, J.T., L.S. Davidow, and D. Warshawsky, *Tsix, a gene antisense to Xist at the X-inactivation centre.* Nat Genet, 1999. 21(4): p. 400-4.
[156] Barakat, T.S., et al., *RNF12 activates Xist and is essential for X chromosome inactivation.* PLoS Genet, 2011. 7(1): p. e1002001.
[157] Jonkers, I., et al., *RNF12 is an X-Encoded dose-dependent activator of X chromosome inactivation.* Cell, 2009. 139(5): p. 999-1011.
[158] Jeon, Y., K. Sarma, and J.T. Lee, *New and Xisting regulatory mechanisms of X chromosome inactivation.* Curr Opin Genet Dev, 2012. 22(2): p. 62-71.
[159] Penny, G.D., et al., *Requirement for Xist in X chromosome inactivation.* Nature, 1996. 379(6561): p. 131-7.
[160] Marahrens, Y., et al., *Xist-deficient mice are defective in dosage compensation but not spermatogenesis.* Genes & Development, 1997. 11(2): p. 156-66.
[161] Wutz, A. and R. Jaenisch, *A shift from reversible to irreversible X inactivation is triggered during ES cell differentiation.* Molecular Cell, 2000. 5(4): p. 695-705.
[162] Ng, K., et al., *A system for imaging the regulatory noncoding Xist RNA in living mouse embryonic stem cells.* Mol Biol Cell, 2011. 22(14): p. 2634-45.
[163] White, W.M., et al., *The spreading of X inactivation into autosomal material of an x;autosome translocation: evidence for a difference*

between *autosomal and X-chromosomal DNA.* American Journal of Human Genetics, 1998. 63(1): p. 20-8.
[164] Riggs, A.D., *DNA methylation and late replication probably aid cell memory, and type I DNA reeling could aid chromosome folding and enhancer function.* Philos Trans R Soc Lond B Biol Sci, 1990. 326(1235): p. 285-97.
[165] Lyon, M.F., *The Lyon and the LINE hypothesis.* Seminars in Cell & Developmental Biology, 2003. 14(6): p. 313-8.
[166] Bailey, J.A., et al., *Molecular evidence for a relationship between LINE-1 elements and X chromosome inactivation: the Lyon repeat hypothesis.* Proceedings of the National Academy of Sciences of the United States of America, 2000. 97(12): p. 6634-9.
[167] Wang, Z., et al., *Evidence of influence of genomic DNA sequence on human X chromosome inactivation.* PLoS Computational Biology, 2006. 2(9): p. e113.
[168] Duret, L., et al., *The Xist RNA gene evolved in eutherians by pseudogenization of a protein-coding gene.* Science, 2006. 312(5780): p. 1653-5.
[169] Chureau, C., et al., *Comparative sequence analysis of the X-inactivation center region in mouse, human, and bovine.* Genome Research, 2002. 12(6): p. 894-908.
[170] Hendrich, B.D., C.J. Brown, and H.F. Willard, *Evolutionary conservation of possible functional domains of the human and murine XIST genes.* Human Molecular Genetics, 1993. 2(6): p. 663-72.
[171] Wutz, A., T.P. Rasmussen, and R. Jaenisch, *Chromosomal silencing and localization are mediated by different domains of Xist RNA.* Nature Genetics, 2002. 30(2): p. 167-74.
[172] Hoki, Y., et al., *A proximal conserved repeat in the Xist gene is essential as a genomic element for X-inactivation in mouse.* Development, 2009. 136(1): p. 139-46.
[173] Caparros, M.L., et al., *Functional analysis of the highly conserved exon IV of XIST RNA.* Cytogenetic and Genome Research, 2002. 99(1-4): p. 99-105.
[174] Hore, T.A., et al., *The region homologous to the X-chromosome inactivation centre has been disrupted in marsupial and monotreme mammals.* Chromosome Res, 2007. 15(2): p. 147-61.
[175] Okamoto, I., et al., *Eutherian mammals use diverse strategies to initiate X-chromosome inactivation during development.* Nature, 2011. 472(7343): p. 370-4.

[176] Migeon, B.R., et al., *Identification of TSIX, encoding an RNA antisense to human XIST, reveals differences from its murine counterpart: implications for X inactivation.* American Journal of Human Genetics, 2001. 69(5): p. 951-60.
[177] Davidow, L.S., et al., *The search for a marsupial XIC reveals a break with vertebrate synteny.* Chromosome Res, 2007. 15(2): p. 137-46.
[178] Shevchenko, A.I., et al., *Genes flanking Xist in mouse and human are separated on the X chromosome in American marsupials.* Chromosome Res, 2007. 15(2): p. 127-36.
[179] Hore, T.A., et al., *The region homologous to the X-chromosome inactivation centre has been disrupted in marsupial and monotreme mammals.* Chromosome Research, 2007. 15(2): p. 147-61.
[180] Shevchenko, A.I., et al., *Genes flanking Xist in mouse and human are separated on the X chromosome in American marsupials.* Chromosome Research, 2007. 15(2): p. 127-36.
[181] Elisaphenko, E.A., et al., *A dual origin of the Xist gene from a protein-coding gene and a set of transposable elements.* PloS One, 2008. 3(6): p. e2521.
[182] Al Nadaf, S., et al., *Activity map of the tammar X chromosome shows that marsupial X inactivation is incomplete and escape is stochastic.* Genome Biol, 2010. 11(12): p. R122.
[183] Grant, J., et al., *Rsx is a metatherian RNA with Xist-like properties in X-chromosome inactivation.* Nature, 2012. 487(7406): p. 254-258.
[184] Clemson, C.M., et al., *The X chromosome is organized into a gene-rich outer rim and an internal core containing silenced nongenic sequences.* Proceedings of the National Academy of Sciences of the United States of America, 2006. 103(20): p. 7688-93.
[185] Kohlmaier, A., et al., *A chromosomal memory triggered by Xist regulates histone methylation in X inactivation.* PLoS Biology, 2004. 2(7): p. e171.
[186] Plath, K., et al., *Role of histone H3 lysine 27 methylation in X inactivation.* Science, 2003. 300(5616): p. 131-5.
[187] Chaumeil, J., et al., *Evolution from XIST-independent to XIST-controlled X-chromosome inactivation: epigenetic modifications in distantly related mammals.* PLoS One, 2011. 6(4): p. e19040.
[188] Graves, J.A., *DNA synthesis in chromosomes of cultured leucocytes from two marsupial species.* Experimental Cell Research, 1967. 46(1): p. 37-57.

[189] Koina, E., et al., *Specific patterns of histone marks accompany X chromosome inactivation in a marsupial.* Chromosome Research, 2009. 17(1): p. 115-26.
[190] Mahadevaiah, S.K., et al., *Key features of the X inactivation process are conserved between marsupials and eutherians.* Current Biology, 2009. 19(17): p. 1478-84.
[191] Rens, W., et al., *Epigenetic modifications on X chromosomes in marsupial and monotreme mammals and implications for evolution of dosage compensation.* Proceedings of the National Academy of Sciences of the United States of America, 2010. 107(41): p. 17657-62.
[192] Hellman, A. and A. Chess, *Gene body-specific methylation on the active X chromosome.* Science, 2007. 315(5815): p. 1141-3.
[193] Bernardino, J., et al., *Common methylation characteristics of sex chromosomes in somatic and germ cells from mouse, lemur and human.* Chromosome Research, 2000. 8(6): p. 513-25.
[194] Rens, W., et al., *Epigenetic modifications on X chromosomes in marsupial and monotreme mammals and implications for evolution of dosage compensation.* Proc Natl Acad Sci U S A, 2010. 107(41): p. 17657-62.
[195] Brockdorff, N., *X-chromosome inactivation: closing in on proteins that bind Xist RNA.* Trends in Genetics, 2002. 18(7): p. 352-8.
[196] Kaslow, D.C. and B.R. Migeon, *DNA methylation stabilizes X chromosome inactivation in eutherians but not in marsupials: evidence for multistep maintenance of mammalian X dosage compensation.* Proceedings of the National Academy of Sciences of the United States of America, 1987. 84(17): p. 6210-4.
[197] Loebel, D.A. and P.G. Johnston, *Analysis of DNase 1 sensitivity and methylation of active and inactive X chromosomes of kangaroos (Macropus robustus) by in situ nick translation.* Chromosoma, 1993. 102(2): p. 81-7.
[198] Loebel, D.A. and P.G. Johnston, *Methylation analysis of a marsupial X-linked CpG island by bisulfite genomic sequencing.* Genome Research, 1996. 6(2): p. 114-23.
[199] Csankovszki, G., A. Nagy, and R. Jaenisch, *Synergism of Xist RNA, DNA methylation, and histone hypoacetylation in maintaining X chromosome inactivation.* The Journal of Cell Biology, 2001. 153(4): p. 773-84.

[200] Murtagh, V.J., et al., *Evolutionary history of novel genes on the tammar wallaby Y chromosome: Implications for sex chromosome evolution.* Genome Res, 2012. 22(3): p. 498-507.
[201] Gribnau, J. and J.A. Grootegoed, *Origin and evolution of X chromosome inactivation.* Curr Opin Cell Biol, 2012. 24(3): p. 397-404.
[202] Sutton, E., et al., *Identification of SOX3 as an XX male sex reversal gene in mice and humans.* J Clin Invest, 2011. 121(1): p. 328-41.
[203] Pask, A.J., et al., *Absence of SOX3 in the developing marsupial gonad is not consistent with a conserved role in mammalian sex determination.* Genesis, 2000. 27(4): p. 145-52.
[204] Cooper, D.W., *Directed genetic change model for X chromosome inactivation in eutherian mammals.* Nature, 1971. 230(5292): p. 292-4.
[205] Takagi, N. and M. Sasaki, *Preferential inactivation of the paternally derived X chromosome in the extraembryonic membranes of the mouse.* Nature, 1975. 256(5519): p. 640-2.
[206] Wake, N., N. Takagi, and M. Sasaki, *Non-random inactivation of X chromosome in the rat yolk sac.* Nature, 1976. 262(5569): p. 580-1.
[207] West, J.D., et al., *Preferential expression of the maternally derived X chromosome in the mouse yolk sac.* Cell, 1977. 12(4): p. 873-82.
[208] Dindot, S.V., et al., *Conservation of genomic imprinting at the XIST, IGF2, and GTL2 loci in the bovine.* Mamm Genome, 2004. 15(12): p. 966-74.
[209] Moreira de Mello, J.C., et al., *Random X inactivation and extensive mosaicism in human placenta revealed by analysis of allele-specific gene expression along the X chromosome.* PLoS One, 2010. 5(6): p. e10947.
[210] Wang, X., et al., *Random X inactivation in the mule and horse placenta.* Genome Research, 2012.
[211] Huynh, K.D. and J.T. Lee, *X-chromosome inactivation: a hypothesis linking ontogeny and phylogeny.* Nat Rev Genet, 2005. 6(5): p. 410-8.
[212] Dementyeva, E.V., et al., *Difference between random and imprinted X inactivation in common voles.* Chromosoma, 2010. 119(5): p. 541-52.
[213] Marahrens, Y., et al., *Xist-deficient mice are defective in dosage compensation but not spermatogenesis.* Genes Dev, 1997. 11(2): p. 156-66.
[214] Okamoto, I., et al., *Evidence for de novo imprinted X-chromosome inactivation independent of meiotic inactivation in mice.* Nature, 2005. 438(7066): p. 369-73.

[215] Kalantry, S., et al., *Evidence of Xist RNA-independent initiation of mouse imprinted X-chromosome inactivation.* Nature, 2009. 460(7255): p. 647-51.
[216] Wang, J., et al., *Imprinted X inactivation maintained by a mouse Polycomb group gene.* Nature genetics, 2001. 28(4): p. 371-5.
[217] Plath, K., et al., *Developmentally regulated alterations in Polycomb repressive complex 1 proteins on the inactive X chromosome.* The Journal of Cell Biology, 2004. 167(6): p. 1025-35.
[218] Migeon, B.R., J. Axelman, and P. Jeppesen, *Differential X reactivation in human placental cells: implications for reversal of X inactivation.* American journal of human genetics, 2005. 77(3): p. 355-64.
[219] Escamilla-Del-Arenal, M., S.T. da Rocha, and E. Heard, *Evolutionary diversity and developmental regulation of X-chromosome inactivation.* Hum Genet, 2011. 130(2): p. 307-27.
[220] Ayoub, N., C. Richler, and J. Wahrman, *Xist RNA is associated with the transcriptionally inactive XY body in mammalian male meiosis.* Chromosoma, 1997. 106(1): p. 1-10.
[221] Turner, J.M., *Meiotic sex chromosome inactivation.* Development, 2007. 134(10): p. 1823-31.
[222] Ohlsson, R., A. Paldi, and J.A. Graves, *Did genomic imprinting and X chromosome inactivation arise from stochastic expression?* Trends Genet, 2001. 17(3): p. 136-41.
[223] Gimelbrant, A., et al., *Widespread monoallelic expression on human autosomes.* Science, 2007. 318(5853): p. 1136-40.

In: Sex Chromosomes: New Research ISBN: 978-1-62417-143-7
Editors: M. D'Aquino and V. Stallone © 2013 Nova Science Publishers, Inc.

Chapter II

Role of Sex Chromosomes in Mammalian Female Fertility

Asma Amleh[1], Bao-Zeng Xu[2] and Teruko Taketo[2,3,][*]
[1]Department of Biology, American University in Cairo, Cairo, Egypt
[2]Urology Research Laboratory, Department of Surgery,
McGill University, Montreal, Quebec, Canada
[3]Department of Biology and Department of Obstetrics and Gynecology,
McGill University, Montreal, Quebec, Canada

Abstract

Oogenesis takes place in the presence of two X-chromosomes in normal mammalian development. While the second X-chromosome is inactivated in all somatic cells, it is reactivated in the female germ cells prior to the onset of meiosis and remains active in the oocyte. The importance of this exception to the X-dosage-compensation rule is understandable but not formally proven. In this review, we discuss the fertility of females carrying atypical sex chromosomes, namely XO and XY. We will briefly touch on human cases, but mainly focus on mouse models. Our laboratory has been studying the mechanism of infertility in the B6.Y^{TIR} sex-reversed female mouse, which carries a single X-chromosome and an intact Y-chromosome. We review the findings from our study of this particular mouse model, with emphasis on the behaviour

---
[*] Corresponding author.

of sex chromosomes during the meiotic progression in the XY oocyte and the consequent ooplasmic defects leading to a failure in the second meiotic division.

Introduction

The sexual differentiation of germ cells follows their gonadal environment, testis or ovary, which is initially determined by the combination of sex chromosomes, XY or XX, in the somatic cells. Thus, spermatogenesis and oogenesis occurs in the presence of XY and XX sex chromosomes, respectively, in normal development. Although the endpoint of gametogenesis is the same for the both sexes, i.e., to provide a haploid set of genomes to offspring, the time course and controlling mechanisms differ tremendously between spermatogenesis and oogenesis. In order to fully understand the role of sex chromosomes in gametogenesis, we need to examine their behaviours in environments other than those of normal XY males or XX females. In this review, we discuss the fertility of females carrying atypical sex chromosomes, namely XO, XY, XXX, XXY, and XYY chromosomes. We briefly discuss human cases, but mainly focus on mouse models. In our laboratory, we have been studying the mechanism of infertility in the B6.Y^{TIR} female mouse, which is sex-reversed despite the presence of an intact Y-chromosome. This mouse model is ideal for comparing the behaviour of X- and Y-chromosomes between the two sexes. We summarize our findings with an emphasis on the behaviour of sex chromosomes during the meiotic progression in the XY oocyte and the consequent ooplasmic defects leading to infertility.

Normal Development of Oocytes in the XX Female

Primordial germ cells (PGCs) originate in the epiblast and migrate into the gonadal primordium prior to sexual differentiation (Tam and Zhou, 1996; Lawson et al., 1999; Molyneaux et al., 2001). Ovarian differentiation is initiated by the activation of genes such as *Wnt4* and *Foxl2*, which antagonize testicular differentiation in gonadal somatic cells, without distinct morphological changes (Ottolenghi et al., 2005; Kim et al., 2006; Maatouk et al., 2008). Instead, most, if not all, germ cells enter meiosis, which characterizes ovarian differentiation in the fetal gonad. Meiosis is essential not only for generating haploid gametes but also for ensuring recombination between homologous chromosomes, resulting in genetically diverse gametes. During the meiotic prophase progression, the paternal and maternal homologous chromosomes including the two X-chromosomes pair and recombine. The second X-chromosome in the XX germ cells is initially inactivated as in any somatic cells, but it is gradually reactivated prior to the onset of meiosis (Monk and McLaren, 1981; Chuva De Sousa Lopes et al., 2008; Sugimoto, 2007). It is reasonable to speculate that the two active X-chromosomes facilitate their pairing and recombination during the meiotic prophase. The oocytes then reach the end of the meiotic prophase, named the diplotene stage, and become arrested at 5-7 months of pregnancy in humans or around the day of delivery in the mouse (Baker, 1963; Speed, 1982; Borum, 1961). Diplotene oocytes become surrounded by granulosa cells and form primordial follicles, which remain at this stage as an oocyte reserve until they are recruited into follicular growth (Bristol-Gould et al., 2006). This resting stage can last for decades in humans or months in the mouse. The oocytes are very active in transcription and protein synthesis during the growth phase, so that they accumulate sufficient cytoplasmic components to carry out subsequent meiotic divisions, fertilization, and early embryonic development, during which transcription has ceased. Therefore, the presence of two X-chromosomes may be beneficial for the accumulation of ooplasmic components. However, the contribution of the second X-chromosome to the developmental competence of oocytes is not fully understood.

XO Females in Humans

XO females can be generated by non-disjunction of sex chromosomes during the first meiotic division in spermatocytes or, less frequently, in oocytes. Another potential cause is the loss of the paternal X-chromosome in the zygote or non-disjunction of sex chromosomes during mitotic divisions in early cleavage-stage embryos. Anomalies of XO females in humans are known as Turners syndrome (TS). The frequency of XO conceptuses is approximately 3%; however, 99% of XO fetuses are spontaneously aborted and the TS disorder is found at the frequency of 1 in 2,000 live-born females (Nielsen and Wohlert, 1991; Stratakis and Rennert, 2005). Less than half of TS cases show a pure 45X karyotype, and the rest are either mosaic or carry a variety of X-chromosome abnormalities and occasionally Y-derived materials (Jacobs et al., 1997; Stratakis and Rennert, 2005). Consequently, the TS phenotype varies, and hidden mosaicism complicates the analysis of the role of the second X-chromosome. Common features of TS include short stature, congenital cardiovascular defects, and metabolic abnormalities. Most TS women are infertile due to the early loss of oocytes (Hreinsson et al., 2002; Modi et al., 2003; Birgit et al., 2009). Occasional cases of pregnancy in TS women have been reported (Tarani et al., 1998; Magee and Hughes, 1998). However, it is difficult to exclude possible mosaicism in these cases. Nonetheless, in those rare cases of pregnancy in TS patients, the rate of miscarriage, stillbirths, or malformed babies is very high (Tarani et al., 1998). Therefore, XO women have, overall, a limited chance to deliver healthy babies.

XO Female Mouse

It is possible to experimentally produce XO females without mosaicism in the mouse. XO female mice were initially found during the breeding of female mice carrying a heterozygous X-autosome translocation, which resulted in the loss of the mutant X-chromosome (Welshons and Russell, 1959; Russel et al., 1959). Similarly, a large inversion in the X-chromosome, named Bare-patches (*Bpa*) or In(X)1H, has generated XO daughters (Phillips et al., 1973; Evans and Phillips, 1975). It remains undetermined whether the mutant X-chromosome was lost during oogenesis or after fertilization (Koehler et al., 2002). Nonetheless, once XO females have been generated, they can produce XO daughters as XO female mice are fertile, unlike humans (Cattanach, 1962). XO females are conveniently distinguished from their XX sisters by introducing a *Tabby* (*Ta*) coat color marker on the X-chromosome from the father (Figure 1A). By alternating breeding with *Ta*-carrier and wild-type males, XO females without *Ta* can be generated. In both above schemes, the resultant XO females carry single X-chromosomes of paternal origin. However, it turned out that the *Ta* mutation causes delayed eyelid opening and incisor eruption, as well as reduced fertility (Deckers and Van der Kroon, 1981; Brook, 1983; Kapalanga and Blecher, 1990). Therefore, a more direct method to identify the XO female, such as karyotyping, performing quantitative PCR of X-chromosome dosage or demonstrating the absence of *Xist* transcripts by RT-PCR, is desirable. Furthermore, the X-chromosome is subjected to genomic imprinting during gametogenesis, and, therefore, XO females carrying the paternal X show severer phenotypes than what is expected from the mere half-dosage of X-chromosome contents (Okamoto, 2004). Their counterparts, XO females carrying the maternal X, have been generated by introducing another mutation on the X-chromosome, named *Patchy fur* (*Paf*), which gives a dominant patchy hair loss phenotype (Lane and Davisson, 1990; Burgoyne and Evans, 2000). In addition to hair loss, hemizygous mutant males have a high incidence of XY non-disjunction during spermatogenesis, producing XO daughters (Figure 1B). This breeding scheme has the advantage that XO females are delivered by normal XX females. Unfortunately, the female *Paf* phenotype disappears on certain genetic backgrounds (e.g., B6), necessitating direct identification of XO females (Alton et al., 2008). Furthermore, the obligatory XX sisters of XO females carry the *Paf* mutation, which reduces fertility (our unpublished observation). It is better to use wild-type XX females at the age and genetic background matching the XO females for comparisons.

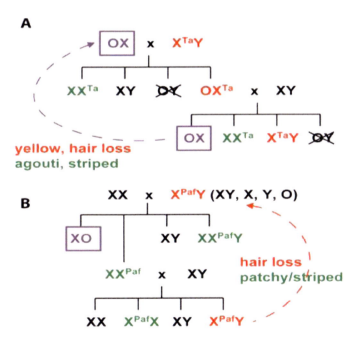

Figure 1. Breeding scheme for XO female production. A. Production of XO females carrying the paternal X. The *Ta* mutation on the X-chromosome is introduced in order to distinguish OX from XX females. B. Production of XO females carrying the maternal X. The *Paf* mutation on the X-chromosome causes X-Y nondisjunction during spermatogenesis and gives a distinct phenotype in its carriers.

Different Effects of the Absence of the Second X-Chromosome in Humans and Mice

XO female mice are viable and healthy unlike the human cases. This difference is mainly explained by the fact that many fewer X-linked genes escape X-inactivation in the mouse as compared to humans; 15% of X-linked genes consistently escape X-inactivation and a further 10% escape in certain tissues or individuals in humans, whereas only 3.3% of X-linked genes escape X-inactivation in the mouse (Fisher et al., 1990; Prothero et al., 2009; Yang et al., 2010). Of the 380 genes located to the X-chromosome, which are inactivated in the mouse, 133 escape X-inactivation in humans. Many such genes have Y-homologues, whose products may have functions similar to those of X-homologues (Prothero et al., 2009). Therefore, the absence of the second X-chromosome can be detrimental in humans, but less so in mice. However, X-chromosome dosage compensation is regulated not only by transcript levels but also by protein levels (Nguyen and Disteche, 2006), and the striking difference between humans and mice remains to be clarified.

Fertility of XO Female Mouse

XO female mice are invariably fertile (Cattanach, 1962; Burgoyne and Baker, 1981; Lyon and Hawker, 1973), making another contrast to human cases. However, it must be noted that the fertility of XO females has been tested on a limited number of genetic backgrounds such as CBA and C3H; XO females may have variable fertility dependent on genetic backgrounds. Furthermore, the XO female mouse has a reduced fertility due to various reasons. In theory, the XO female produces zygotes of four genotypes, XO, YO, XX, and XY. Because of the loss of YO embryos, a 25% reduction of litter size and equal proportions of XO and XX females would be anticipated if the single X-chromosome were to be segregated randomly during meiotic divisions. However, XO female offspring are always smaller in number than expected. In addition, the XO female has a smaller oocyte reserve and, hence, a shorter reproductive life compared to the XX female. We will discuss these points in more detail in the following sections.

Influence of the Genetic Background

The genetic background may influence these factors which can affect the fertility of XO females: 1) the ratio of mature oocytes missing the X-chromosome after the first meiotic division, 2) the survival and fertility of oocytes missing the X-chromosome, 3) the survival of XO embryos in the uterus (In this case, both the mother and the father contribute to the genetic background of embryos), and 4) the number and retention of oocytes in the XO female. In previous studies, however, these factors were not individually analyzed. Instead, we provide information in the following paragraph as to the influence of the genetic background on the rate of XO offspring production, which is the sum of the first three factors.

The original XO females carrying the paternal X were identified on a mixed background, which was switched to the inbred CBA background (Cattanach, 1962). In this genetic background, approximately 25% of female offspring were XO. Similarly, a 26% rate of XO female production was reported for the cross between the In(X)/X female and the wild-type male on the Swiss albino background (Speed, 1986) and 17% on the (B6.DBA)F1 background (Jamieson et al., 1998). On the other hand, by crossing the wild-type female with the *Paf*-carrier male, 12-19% of daughters were XO females carrying the maternal X on the C3H background (Lyon and Hawker, 1973; Jamieson et al., 1998), and this ratio decreased on the outbred MF1 background (Burgoyne and Evans, 2000). In our laboratory, we transferred the *Paf* mutation from the C3H to B6 background by repeated backcrosses, and obtained a 22-23 % rate of XO females up to the 8th backcross generation; however, the ratio of XO offspring dramatically dropped to near zero after further backcrosses (unpublished). It is also reported that the B6 background leads to a high rate of the loss of XO embryos carrying the paternal X (Hunt, 1991). We have confirmed that at similar backcross generations, XO females carrying the maternal X are born from *Paf*-carrier fathers, but they have never produced XO daughters carrying the paternal X by mating with wild-type males (unpublished).

The genetic background appears to affect the reproductive life span of XO females; fertility over 10 months was reported for the XO females carrying the paternal X on a mixed genetic background (Lyon and Hawker, 1973), whereas no pregnancy was recognized over 6 months for the XO females carrying the maternal X on the B6 background (Hunt, 1991)(our unpublished observation).

Deficit in XO Embryos

The deficit in XO embryos can be attributed to two mechanisms: preferential retention of the single X-chromosome in the mature oocyte and excessive loss of XO embryos in utero. Non-random segregation of X-chromosomes was suggested by some authors (Kaufman, 1972; Luthardt, 1976; Xu et al., 2012; Sakurada et al., 1994), but not confirmed by others (Brook, 1983). On the other hand, retarded development of XO embryos carrying the paternal X has been consistently observed (Burgoyne et al., 1983; Burgoyne and Biggers, 1976; Burgoyne and Rastan, 1991; Thornhill and Burgoyne, 1993; Jamieson et al., 1998) although normal development of XO embryos was also reported (Omoe and Endo, 1993). It has been hypothesized that since the paternal X has been imprinted during spermatogenesis to become preferentially inactivated in the extraembryonic tissue, it may be less capable than the maternal X in providing the appropriate dosage of X-linked activity. However, this hypothesis contradicts the recent finding that haploid embryos carrying the paternal X develop normally up to the blastocyst stage (Yang et al., 2012). Alternatively, the paternal X may be less vigorous to support the placental development (Ishikawa et al., 2003). Development of XO embryos carrying the maternal X appears to be normal, but these cases have not been robustly studied (Thornhill and Burgoyne, 1993; Jamieson et al., 1998; Burgoyne and Evans, 2000; Alton et al., 2008). *Xlr3b* and *Xlr4b/c* are the only genes known to be differentially expressed from the maternal X in the brain of XO females (so as XY females) (Davies et al., 2005; Raefski and O'Neill, 2005). Interestingly, *Xlr3* is also expressed in ovaries, and *Xlr* genes have homology with *Scp3*, which is essential for the meiotic prophase progression in the oocyte. Further studies are awaited to clarify the difference between XO females with the maternal X and those with the paternal X.

Excessive Loss of Oocytes in XO Females

XO females, regardless of the parental origin of the X, show a shorter reproductive life span compared to their XX littermates (Lyon and Hawker, 1973; Xu et al., 2012; Burgoyne and Baker, 1981). One explanation is an excessive loss of oocytes during the meiotic prophase progression in the perinatal ovary (Burgoyne and Baker, 1985). Consequently, XO females have a smaller oocyte reserve than XX females, and prematurely end their reproductive life (Burgoyne and Baker, 1981; Xu et al., 2012). It has been proposed that the lack of a pairing partner for the single X-chromosome leads to oocyte demise triggered by a pachytene checkpoint surveillance mechanism, although some XO oocytes do survive by forming a non-homologous association with the X itself or with an autosome (Speed, 1986). Alternatively, an unsynapsed X-chromosome is silenced by a mechanism called "meiotic silencing of unsynapsed chromosome (MSUC)", and XO oocytes die or survive depending on the silenced genes (Baarends et al., 2005; Mahadevaiah et al., 2008; Burgoyne et al., 2009; Kouznetsova et al., 2009; Turner et al., 2005). The link between X-chromosome asynapsis and oocyte demise remains to be established.

XY Females in Humans

In normal development, a single exon gene *SRY* on the Y-chromosome is activated in the XY gonadal primordium, and initiates a cascade of molecular and morphological events leading to testicular differentiation (Sinclair et al., 1990; Koopman et al., 1991). In theory, therefore, the disturbance of any of the genes involved in this process would result in partial or complete sex-reversal. In the absence of testicular differentiation, ovarian differentiation is initiated in the XY gonad, allowing the development of a female phenotype. Anomalies of XY females in humans are known as Swyer syndrome (Behzadian et al., 1991). 15-20% of XY sex reversal can be attributed to *SRY* mutations, including point mutations, frame-shifts and deletions (Cameron and Sinclair, 1997; Lim et al., 1998). *SRY* encodes a DNA binding protein containing a HMG-box motif (Sinclair et al., 1990). Consequently, mutations of *SRY* in its DNA binding-motif or mutations of the genes encoding calmodulin or β-importin, which are required for SRY nuclear localization, block SRY actions and result in sex reversal (Harley et al., 1992; Harley et al., 2003; Kaur et al., 2010; Sim et al., 2005). The direct target of SRY is *SOX9*, which shares the DNA binding motif with *SRY* (Meyer et al., 1997; Foster et al., 1994; Wagner et al., 1994). Heterozygous mutations of *SOX9* lead to a congenital bone and cartilage malformation named Campomelic dysplasia, which is frequently associated with XY sex reversal (Cameron and Sinclair, 1997). The cause of XY sex reversal in many other cases remains an enigma (Kwok et al., 1996; Cotinot et al., 2002; Vaiman and Pailhoux, 2000). It must be noted that a mutation of either *SRY* or *SOX9* can be identified in both a fertile father and his XY daughter(s) within a family, suggesting that the genetic cause of sex reversal has conditional penetrance, which makes the analysis of a genetic cause challenging (Cameron and Sinclair, 1997; Lim et al., 1998).

XY women are exclusively infertile. A rare fertile case was found in a woman who was mosaic, carrying predominantly the XY karyotype in the ovary, but she transmitted only the X-chromosome to her XY daughter (Dumic et al., 2008). 7-10% of XY females have a risk of developing gonadoblastoma (Uehara et al., 1999; Lau, 1999; Manuel et al., 1976; Gravholt et al., 2000). Therefore, gonads are surgically removed in most cases of XY sex reversal when identified. Oocyte donation is the only option for these women in order to conceive babies (Frydman et al., 1988; Tulic et al., 2011).

XY Female Mouse

In addition to *Sry*, over ten genes have been identified to play critical roles in testicular differentiation in the mouse; their functional deletion results in sex reversal in the XY gonad. These genes can be divided into five groups according to their positions in the testis-determining pathway: 1. those required for gonadal formation of both sexes (e.g., *Wt1*, *Sf1*), 2. those that affect *Sry* expression (e.g., *Wt1*, *Fog2*, *Gata4*), 3. those that modify SRY actions (*Sf1*, *Sox9*), 4. those that transmit the SRY action into the cellular and morphological differentiation of testicular components (e.g., *Sox9*, *Fgf9*, *Dhh*), and 5. those that stabilize *Sox9* expression (e.g., *Fgf9*, *Sf1*, *Pgd2*). We do not intend to repeat the information which is available in other reviews (Brennan and Capel, 2004; Kashimada and Koopman, 2010; Sekido and Lovell-Badge, 2008; Wilhelm et al., 2007; Schartl, 2004; Park and Jameson, 2005). However, we emphasize a couple of points which are relevant to the study of XY female fertility. First, a complete sex reversal by autosomal gene mutations is rare since the XY ovary develops only when testicular components are absent or limited to a small proportion (Mullen and Whitten, 1971; Singh et al., 1987). Second, all autosomal genes involved in testicular differentiation are expressed in other cell types and organs; these mutations lead to multifactorial defects, and, therefore, the long term consequence of sex reversal, such as fertility, has not been tested except for a conditional *Sox9* null mutation (Lavery et al., 2011). Thus, XY female mouse models for studying the influence of the Y-chromosome on female fertility are limited to those with impaired SRY functions (Table 1).

Fertility of XY female mice depends on the cause of sex reversal as well as the genetic background. When sex reversal is caused by the deletion of a Y-chromosome region harbouring *Sry*, the resultant XY^{Tdy1} female on a mixed genetic background has severely reduced fertility; nonetheless, it occasionally produces offspring (Lovell-Badge and Robertson, 1990).

A slightly better fertility was reported for the XY^{Tdy1} female on the outbred MF1 background after delivered by XXY ^{Tdy1} females (Mahadevaiah et al., 1993) By contrast, when most copies of the repetitive *Rbmy* sequence on the Y-chromosome have been deleted, the *Sry* sequence remains intact, but its expression during gonadal differentiation is repressed, and sex reversal ensues. These XY^{dl} females are as fertile as XO females on the MF1 background (Capel et al., 1993).

In the XY females, named B6.Y^{POS} or B6.Y^{TIR}, the *Sry* gene is intact and expressed during gonadal differentiation, and yet testicular differentiation fails. These XY females are sterile except for one litter at an early stage of backcross generation (Eicher et al., 1982; Taketo-Hosotani et al., 1989; Lee and Taketo, 1994; Taketo et al., 2005). (We will discuss these cases of sex reversal in more detail.) In the XY female mouse, in which *Sox9* has been conditionally deleted from gonadal somatic cells while the *Sry* gene remains intact, low levels of fertility on a mixed background have been reported (Lavery et al., 2011).

Thus, the physical presence of the Y-chromosome does not prevent female fertility, but the structure or gene expression of the Y-chromosome appears to have a critical influence on female fertility.

Table 1. Cause and degree of fertility in female mice carrying atypical sex chromosomes

Sex chromosomes	X-Ch	Y-Ch	Sry	Genetic background	Fertility
XX	2	absent	absent	any	++
XO	1	absent	absent	CBA, C3H, B6, MF1, mixed	+
XY^{Tdy1}	1	*Sry* deletion	absent	MF1, mixed	±
XY^{dl}	1	*Rbmy* deletion	repressed	MF1, mixed	+
B6.Y^{TIR}	1	intact	expressed	B6	-
XY^{SOX9}	1	intact	expressed	mixed	±

Mechanism of Sex Reversal in B6.Y^{POS} and B6.Y^{TIR} Mice

We have been particularly interested in the B6.Y^{TIR} mouse since sex reversal occurs in the presence of all intact chromosomes including X and Y. Therefore, this mouse model provides an opportunity for studying the role of an intact Y-chromosome in female fertility. B6.Y^{POS} and B6.Y^{TIR} mice have been generated by transferring the Y-chromosomes of *Mus musculus domesticus* local variants, caught in Poschiavinus Valley, Switzerland (POS) and Tirano, Italy (TIR), respectively, onto the B6 genetic background by repeated backcrosses (Eicher et al., 1982; Nagamine et al., 1987a). After the eighth backcross generation, all XY progeny fail to develop normal testes and instead develop ovaries or ovotestes in early fetal life. Since the Y^{POS}- or Y^{TIR}-chromosome can initiate normal testicular differentiation on all but the B6 genetic background, whereas the B6 genetic background can support normal testicular differentiation initiated by the Y-chromosomes of B6 and many other strains, the genetic mechanism of sex reversal in B6.Y^{POS} and B6.Y^{TIR} mice can be attributed to an incompatibility between the Y-chromosome of POS/TIR and the autosomal gene(s) of B6 (Eicher et al., 1982; Nagamine et al., 1987b). It is now evident that *Sry* is the gene on the Y-chromosome involved in this manner of sex reversal (Eicher et al., 1995) although the molecular mechanism of sex reversal remains to be clarified. On the other hand, the autosomal genes responsible for this sex reversal have been linked to some areas of Chromosomes 2 and 4, but remain unidentified (Eicher and Washburn, 1986).

Low expression levels of *Sry* are at least partly responsible for sex reversal in B6.Y^{POS} and B6.Y^{TIR} mice. It has been reported by various laboratories that *Sry* transcript levels in the gonadal primordium of B6.Y^{POS} or B6.Y^{TIR} mouse are lower than those of many other mouse strains (Nagamine et al., 1999; Eicher et al., 1982; Lee and Taketo, 2001; Albrecht et al., 2003). Furthermore, overexpression of an *Sry* transgene of the Y^{POS} origin prevents sex reversal in the B6.Y^{POS} mouse, confirming the quantitative nature of sex reversal mechanism (Albrecht et al., 2003; Eicher et al., 1995). However, this mechanism alone is not sufficient to explain the cause of sex reversal since both *Sry* transcript and protein levels in the gonadal primordium of the normal B6.XY strain are as low as those of the B6.Y^{TIR} strain (Lee and Taketo, 1994; Lee and Taketo, 2001; Park et al., 2011; Taketo et al., 2005) (Figure 2). There must be a functional difference in the *Sry* products of the Y^{B6}-origin and those of the Y^{POS}- or Y^{TIR}-origin. Indeed, a polymorphic difference in the *Sry* open-reading frame makes the SRY protein encoded on the Y^{TIR}-chromosome much shorter than that encoded on the Y^{B6}-chromosome (Coward et al., 1994; Taketo et al., 2005). However, the short form of SRY can initiate normal testicular differentiation in many mouse strains such as FVB and CD1. We have hypothesized that the short SRY protein, in combination with its low expression levels, reduces the efficiency of SRY action; consequently, *Sox9* upregulation is delayed while the ovarian differentiation pathway takes over (Park et al., 2008). This hypothesis is consistent with findings by other investigators (Dubin et al., 1995; Moreno-Mendoza et al., 2004; Bullejos and Koopman, 2005). We must emphasize that the *Sox9* expression pattern in the B6.Y^{TIR} gonad is complex; despite the delay in the onset, SOX9 proteins are expressed in the entire region of all gonads and then disappear, allowing ovarian differentiation, in either the entire region or only on both poles (Park et al., 2008). Therefore, the stabilization of *Sox9* expression is the key to success of testicular differentiation in the B6.Y^{TIR} gonad. It remains to be addressed whether these early molecular events, i.e., the expression of SRY and SOX9 in somatic cells during gonadal sex differentiation, has any impact on later ovarian development and fertility.

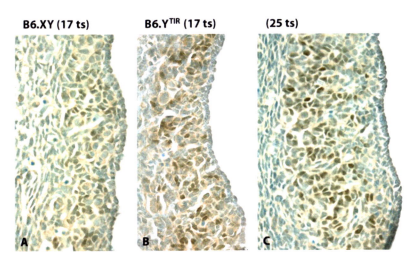

Figure 2. Immunocytochemical detection of SRY proteins (brown) in B6.XY (A) and B6.Y^{TIR} (B and C) gonadal primordia at embryonic day 11. Developmental stage of each fetus was determined by the number of tail-somites (ts). In all histological sections, gonadal primordium and mesonephros are positioned on the right and left, respectively. Counterstained with methyl green. Note the nuclear localization of SRY proteins in the entire region of both B6.XY and B6.Y^{TIR} gonads.

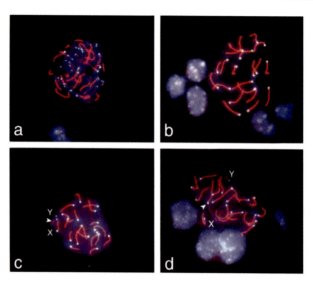

Figure 3. Sex chromosome pairing during the meiotic prophase progression. Immunofluorescence staining of synaptonemal complex (SC) proteins (red) and centromeres (green) with DAPI nuclear staining (blue). (a) XX oocyte at the zygotene stage. Partial pairing between homologous chromosomes is seen by the thickening of SC staining. Most of the centromeres are not yet paired. (b) XX oocyte at the pachytene stage. 20 discreet SC cores between homologous chromosomes and centromeres are seen. (c) XY spermatocyte at the pachytene stage from a B6.Y^{TIR} male, which was not sex reversed. In addition to 19 autosome pairs, the X- and Y-chromosomes are paired at their termini (arrowhead). (d) XY oocyte at the pachytene stage from a B6.Y^{TIR} female. The Y-chromosomes is left alone while the single X-chromosome (arrowhead) is tangled with autosomal pairs. From (Amleh et al., 2000).

Cause of Infertility in the B6.Y^{TIR} Female Mouse

More than half of B6.Y^{TIR} gonads develop into ovaries, in which germ cells enter meiosis and go through the meiotic prophase (Taketo-Hosotani et al., 1989; Alton et al., 2008; Amleh et al., 1996). The X- and Y-chromosomes do not pair in the XY oocyte, unlike in the XY spermatocyte (Figure 3), but a considerable number of XY oocytes survive to complete the meiotic prophase and form follicles (Taketo-Hosotani et al., 1989; Alton et al., 2008) (Figure 4). The B6.Y^{TIR} mouse carrying bilateral ovaries develops a female phenotype (named XY female hereafter), which is anatomically indistinguishable from that of its XX sisters. At young ages, the XY ovary is full of follicles (Alton et al., 2008; Amleh et al., 1996) (Figure 4). The rate of follicular development and atresia in the XY ovary is comparable with those in the XX ovary, except that preovulatory follicles are rarely seen in the XY ovary (Amleh et al., 1996; Wong et al., 2000). Nonetheless, the XY female does not produce oocytes which are competent for embryonic development. The XY female rapidly loses oocytes with age, and very few are left in its ovaries by 2 months after birth (Taketo-Hosotani et al., 1989). Consequently, adult XY females have normal mating behaviors, but lack estrous cyclicity and never produce offspring by natural mating. On the other hand, if XY females have received XX ovarian grafts, they can get pregnant, deliver and nurse pups (Marmolejo-Valencia et al., 1999). Therefore, the primary cause of infertility in the XY female is in its ovaries. In the following sections, we summarize our studies in quest of the cause of infertility in the B6.Y^{TIR} ovary.

Excessive Loss of XY Oocytes

The onset and progression of the meiotic prophase in the XY ovary is comparable to that in the XX ovary up to its embryonic day (ED) 16 (Park and Taketo, 2003; Taketo-Hosotani et al., 1989). However, the oocytes that enter meiosis early in the XY ovary fail to complete the meiotic prophase and disappear entirely from the central region by ED19 (usually the day of delivery). On the other hand, oocytes which enter meiosis later, being concentrated in the cortical region, reach the end of the meiotic prophase and contribute to follicle formation. Overall, the number of follicles in the XY neonatal ovary is smaller than that in the XX or XO ovary. Since X- and Y-chromosomes do not pair in the XY oocyte during the meiotic prophase, the excessive loss of oocytes in the XY ovary can be attributed to the same mechanisms as those discussed for the XO oocyte. However, the early and selective loss of oocytes in the central region does not occur in the XO ovary (Alton et al., 2008). Therefore, the Y-chromosome appears to add a disadvantage on the survival of XY oocytes. We cannot exclude the possibility that longer expression of SRY and SOX9 in the central region of the gonadal primordium, albeit temporarily, makes the somatic environment in this region hostile to the oocyte (Alton et al., 2008; Taketo et al., 2005; Park et al., 2011). In the XX ovary, the oocytes in the central region are postnatally eliminated following follicular growth, presumably due to an insufficient supply of gonadotropins. Therefore, the prenatal loss of oocytes in the central region cannot directly account for the rapid loss of all oocytes in the prepubertal XY female.

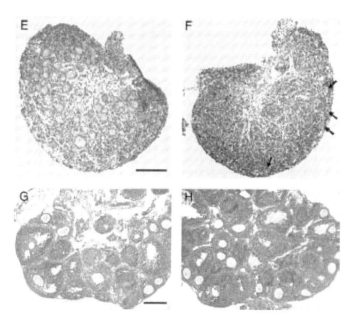

Figure 4. XX (E and G) and XY (F and H) ovaries at 5 days (E and F) and 28 days (G and H) after birth, stained with hematoxylin and eosin. Arrows (F) indicate oocytes near the surface epithelium. Bar (E and G) indicates 200 μm (same for F and H, respectively). From (Alton et al., 2008).

Endocrine Features in the XY Ovary

The XY ovary at one day after birth can convert pregnenolone to progesterone and testosterone to estradiol in culture with an equal efficiency to the XX ovary (Villalpando et al., 1993). Testosterone levels are undetectable in both genotypes of ovaries, confirming that the XY ovary is endocrinologically sex-reversed. At 14 days after birth, the endocrine profile of the XY ovary becomes abnormal; progesterone production is higher while testosterone and estradiol production is lower compared to the XX ovary. Furthermore, testosterone production is drastically increased by the addition of gonadotropins in the XX ovary, but not in the XY ovary. Distribution of 3β-hydroxysteroid dehydrogenase (3β-HSD), which is required for progesterone synthesis, also differs; it is highly concentrated in growing follicles and the interstitium of the central region in the XX ovary whereas it is in the epithelial cords which have developed in the follicle-free central region in the XY ovary. By 35 days after birth, the levels of all steroids produced by the XY ovary become consistently 60% of those by the XX ovary. These lower levels of steroid production can be attributed to a smaller number of follicles. However, the lack of responsiveness to gonadotropins in the production of progesterone and testosterone persists in the XY ovary. By contrast, the conversion of testosterone to estradiol increases in response to gonadotropins to a similar extent in XX and XY ovaries. LH receptors are also similarly distributed in XX and XY ovaries, except for their absence in the rare preovulatory follicles in the XY ovary (Amleh et al., 1996). In conclusion, the endocrine feature of the XY ovary shows abnormality during development, but establishes a normal balance overall by the pre-pubertal ages.

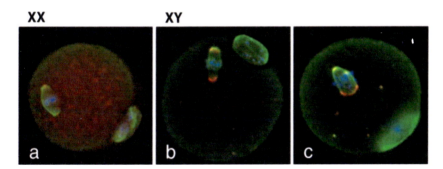

Figure 5. Second meiotic spindles in the oocytes after maturation in vitro. (a) The spindle is symmetrical and parallel to the ooplasmic membrane in the oocyte from an XX female. (b) The spindle is symmetrical but with wider poles and positioned perpendicular to the ooplasmic membrane in the oocyte from an XY female. (c) The spindle is asymmetrical with a wider pole in the oocyte from an XY female. From (Obata et al., 2008).

Failure in the Second Meiotic Division

Although the young XY female ovulates, the number of ovulated eggs is limited, and they do not develop beyond the 2-cell stage after fertilization in vivo or vitro (Merchant-Larios et al., 1994; Taketo-Hosotani et al., 1989). To avoid problems associated with ovulation, we collected fully-grown (or GV-stage) oocytes surrounded by cumulus cells (named COC) from antral follicles and let them mature in vitro. The oocytes from XX and XY ovaries resume meiotic progression, go through the first meiotic division, and reach the second meiotic metaphase (MII) at comparable rates (Amleh et al., 1996; Villemure et al., 2007; Obata et al., 2008). However, the MII-oocytes from XY females contain aberrant spindles with loosely aligned metaphase chromosomes, diffuse poles, and a perpendicular orientation instead of a parallel one (Villemure et al., 2007; Obata et al., 2008) (Figure 5). After fertilization or activation, these oocytes exhibit Ca^{2+} oscillations, but their sister chromatids fail to segregate in their majority (Villemure et al., 2007). The fertilized oocytes eventually enter the interphase but reach the 2-cell stage at a much lower rate than those of control XX females and rarely reach the blastocyst stage (Amleh et al., 1996). Thus, the oocytes of XY females are competent for meiotic maturation but incompetent for embryonic development largely due to a defect in the second meiotic division.

Ooplasmic Defects Responsible for the Second Meiotic Division

In order to determine whether the failure in the second meiotic division can be attributed to the nucleus or cytoplasm, we transferred the nucleus of an XY oocyte into an enucleated XX oocyte at the GV-stage and allowed the reconstituted oocyte to mature in vitro (Obata et al., 2008) (Figure 6A). The reconstituted oocyte, which carries the nucleus from the XY oocyte, assembles a normal second meiotic spindle, completes embryonic development, and transmits the maternal Y-chromosome into its offspring. These results clearly indicate that the nucleus of the XY oocyte can generate healthy offspring as long as proper ooplasm is provided. We also performed nuclear transfers at the MII-stage by using ovulated eggs as recipients (Figure 6B). The second meiotic spindle is properly reassembled in the nucleus from an XY oocyte after incubation for only one hour, confirming that aberrant spindles can be attributed to ooplasmic defects in the XY oocyte. Nonetheless, a smaller percentage of reconstituted oocytes succeed in embryonic development, compared to those aided by nuclear transfer at the GV-stage. We tested the nature of the ooplasmic defect by transferring 5-20% in volume of the cytoplasm from an XX oocyte into an XY oocyte at the GV-stage or vise versa, and found that the second meiotic spindle assembly in the XY oocyte improves with the supplementation of normal ooplasm, but a reciprocal combination has no effect (unpublished). We speculate that the cytoplasm of the XY oocyte is deficient in the components which are essential for the second meiotic spindle assembly and subsequent chromosome segregation.

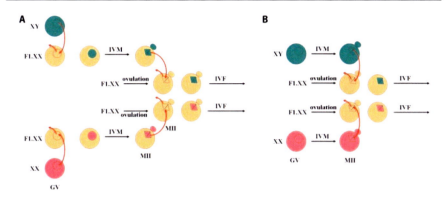

Figure 6. Experimental design of nuclear transfer. A. Nucleus of XX or XY oocyte at the GV-stage was transferred into an enucleated GV-stage oocyte of an F1.XX female, and matured in vitro. The nucleus of a mature oocyte was transferred into an enucleated oocyte ovulated by an F1.XX female. B. XX or XY oocytes at the GV-stage were matured in vitro. The nucleus of a mature oocyte was transferred into an enucleated oocyte ovulated by an F1.XX female. All reconstructed oocytes were subjected to IVF by sperm from F1.XY males.

Defective Components in the XY Oocyte

We compared the gene expression profiles in fully grown oocytes collected from XY ovaries with those from XX ovaries by cDNA microarray (Xu et al., 2012). Four Y-encoded, eight X-encoded, and 161 autosomal genes show higher transcript levels, whereas 77 X-encoded and 408 autosomal genes show lower transcript levels in XY oocytes than in XX oocytes by at least 2-fold. We compared the transcript levels of selected genes by semi-quantitative RT-PCR (sqRT-PCR). In these studies, we included the XO oocytes carrying the maternal X-chromosomes. We confirmed that Y-encoded *Eif2s3y*, *Ddx3y*, *Ubely1*, and *Uty* are expressed at high levels and *Rbmy*, *Ssty*, *Ups9y*, and *Zfy1* are expressed at much lower levels only in XY oocytes. We initially anticipated a dosage dependence of X-encoded gene transcript levels in XY and XO oocytes. However, all genes tested show comparable transcript levels between XX and XO oocytes, indicating that the storage of mRNAs is well adjusted in these oocytes. By comparison, many X-encoded and autosomal genes show higher or lower transcript levels in XY oocytes, suggesting that the processing or accumulation of mRNAs is altered in XY oocytes. Such differences in mRNA profiles may explain the fertility of XO oocytes and infertility of XY oocytes.

Defects in the XY Oocyte Reflected in Its Neighboring Follicular Cells

The oocyte develops intimate and interdependent association with its surrounding granulosa cells during folliculogensis (Brower and Schultz, 1982; Buccione et al., 1990; Anderson and Albertini, 1976). Through gap junctions, follicular cells provide growth factors, nutrients, and other unidentified factors that affect oocyte growth and maturation, whereas the oocyte secretes factors such as GDF9 and BMP15 that regulate follicular cell proliferation, differentiation, and functions (Buccione et al., 1990; Eppig, 2005; Sugiura and Eppig, 2005). Our results show that the defects in the XY oocyte are associated with defects in its surrounding cumulus cells (unpublished). We first found that the fully-grown oocyte of the XY female contains abnormally high transcript levels of *Amy2a5* and *Epas1* (also known as *Hif1a*), a sign of low glucose and oxygen supplies (Xu et al., 2012). We then found that the transcript levels of *Pfkp*, *Pkm2*, and *Ldh1* involved in glycolysis are lower in the cumulus cells surrounding the XY oocyte compared to those surrounding the XX oocyte. Glycolysis provides the substrates for ATP production, which is essential for many physiological events including spindle assembly in the oocyte. We found that the ATP content in XY oocytes is lower than that in XX oocytes at both GV- and MII-stages (unpublished). We hypothesize that altered gene expression in the oocyte exacerbates its cytoplasmic defects, including low ATP content, by affecting its neighboring follicular cell functions through bi-directional communication.

To determine whether interdependent negative effects are initiated by the XY oocyte or its surrounding XY somatic cells, we constructed mouse chimeras by aggregating 8-cell stage embryos from the B6 x B6.Y^{TIR} cross and those from the BALB/c strain. All B6.Y^{TIR} ↔ XX chimeric females composed of up to 95% XY cells produce offspring derived from XX oocytes (Amleh and Taketo, 1998). These results suggest that the XY oocyte is intrinsically defective whereas the presence of XY somatic cells in the chimeric ovary allows the development of fertile XX oocytes. This conclusion is further supported by the experiments in which COCs of XY ovaries were cultured for 20 hr in the presence of milrinone, which maintains the oocyte arrested at the GV-stage. The glycolysis gene transcript levels in the cumulus cells returned to the same levels as in the COCs of XX ovaries (unpublished). The results of our studies together suggest that the XY oocyte becomes defective in its cytoplasm in early development, probably through the expression of Y-encoded genes, and fails to support the full differentiation of follicular cells, which in turn exacerbate cytoplasmic defects in the XY oocyte.

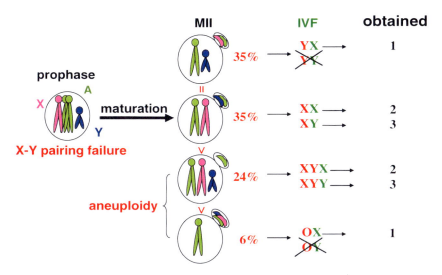

Figure 7. Hypothetical inheritance of sex chromosomes from the XY oocyte by nuclear transfer and fertilization. The unpaired X- and Y-chromosomes are segregated independently but not randomly (subjected to a meiotic drive) at the first meiotic division. The average % of oocytes of each genotype is shown next to the MII-oocyte. The sex chromosome of maternal origin and that of paternal origin in embryos are shown in red and green, respectively. Actual number of pups, theoretically developed from these embryos, is given at the right. No XY progeny carrying a single maternal Y was obtained, but one XY progeny carrying two maternal Ys is included as YX. Based on (Villemure et al., 2007; Obata et al., 2008).

Behavior of the Y-chromosome in Oogenesis

The nucleus of the XY oocyte can produce offspring as long as proper cytoplasm is provided (Obata et al., 2008). It is worth addressing the fate of the X- and Y-chromosomes in the oocyte and through embryonic development. We have shown that the X- and Y-chromosomes never pair during the meiotic prophase (Alton et al., 2008; Amleh et al., 2000) (Figure 3). Consequently, X- and Y-chromosomes are segregated independently during the first meiotic division (Villemure et al., 2007; Amleh et al., 2000). However, their distribution is not random; 65% of MII-oocytes retain single sex chromosomes, equally X or Y, 24% retain both X and Y, and the rest retain none (Figure 7). After nuclear transfer and fertilization, the karyotype of offspring faithfully reflects this distribution of sex chromosomes although the sample size is limited; XXY and XYY (both are males on an F1 background) appear as frequently as XX and XY whereas XO offspring are found less frequently (Obata et al., 2008). We have obtained an XYY progeny carrying two maternal Ys but no XY progeny carrying a single maternal Y. We included this example as XY with a maternal Y, but we need further studies to confirm whether or not the XY embryo carrying a single maternal Y is viable. Overall, it appears that sex chromosome aneuploidy does not block oogenesis or embryonic development except that YY and YO embryos do not survive beyond early cleavage stages.

XXX, XXY and XYY Females

XXX females are common in humans, reported to be 1 out of every 1,000 females (Nielsen and Wohlert, 1991). Nondisjunction of X-chromosomes at the first meiotic division in the oocyte is mainly responsible for the genesis of human XXX females (MacDonald et al., 1994; May et al., 1990). XXX women have normal fertility and rarely generate offspring with sex chromosome aneuploidy, which is explained by the loss of the third X-chromosome in germ cells whereas all but one X-chromosome are inactivated in somatic cells (Hall et al., 2006). Because of the largely normal phenotype, many XXX women probably remain unrecognized. By contrast, XXY and XYY females are rare in humans because the Y-chromosome usually makes the XXY or XYY individual develop as a male. On the other hand, it is possible to experimentally produce XXY, and XYY females in the mouse (Mahadevaiah et al., 1993). XXX females are difficult to obtain in the mouse since the presence of an extra maternal X causes early death of XXX and XXY embryos (Shao and Takagi, 1990). This species difference is explained by the stability of genomic imprinting on the maternal X; which is more resistant to inactivation due to fast implantation and embryonic development in the mouse. It has been reported that the XXY female shows much better fertility than the XY female, suggesting that the lack of the second X is the major cause of poor fertility of the XY female (Mahadevaiah et al., 1993) (In these experiments, sex reversal was induced due to the deletion of an *Sry*-encompassing region on the Y-chromosome). However, the XYY female has poorer fertility than the XY female, suggesting that the Y-chromosome, in addition, exerts negative effects on female fertility.

Summary and Future Directions

In *Mus musculus*, the absence of the second X-chromosome reduces female fertility, and the presence of the Y-chromosome further reduces it. We have presented data to support the hypothesis that the cause of infertility in the B6.Y^{TIR} female mouse is intrinsic to its ovary, likely mediated by the expression of Y-encoded genes in the oocyte. Furthermore, the defective oocyte influences the surrounding follicular cells, which in turn exacerbate the cytoplasmic defects in the oocyte. Consequently, the second metaphase spindle formation is disturbed, but the nucleus of the XY oocyte per se maintains the ability to produce healthy offspring after fertilization. Unfortunately, the fertility of other types of XY females has not been studied to the same extent. It is conceivable that the B6 genetic background is particularly vulnerable to the absence of the second X-chromosome or the presence of the Y-chromosome. Nonetheless, the behaviour of the Y-chromosome in the oocytes of the B6.Y^{TIR} female mouse promotes our understanding of the role of sex chromosomes in female fertility. XY females are fertile in some rodent species such as *Akodon* (Hoekstra and Hoekstra, 2001; Hoekstra, 2003; Espinosa and Vitullo, 1996). Therefore, there appears to be no evolutionary force to make the XY female infertile. It remains to be determined what kind of disadvantages the Y-chromosome imposes on female fertility in mammalian species.

Acknowledgment

We would like to thank all past and present members of Taketo's laboratory as well as our collaborators, particularly Drs. C. Nagamine (Stanford University), H. Merchant-Larios (National University of Mexico), Y-F.C. Lau (University of California, San Francisco), and Y. Obata (Tokyo University of Agriculture). We also thank Dr. P. Burgoyne (NIMR, Mill Hill, London) for his critical reading of the initial manuscript. A part of these studies were supported by grants from Medical Research Council of Canada and Canadian Institute for Health Research to T.T.

References

Albrecht, K.H., Young, M., Wahsburn, L.L., and Eicher, E.M. (2003). Sry Expression level and protein isoform differences play a role in abnormal testis development in C57BL/6J mice carrying certain *Sry* alleles. *Genet. Soc. Am.* 164, 277-288.

Alton, M., Lau, M.P., Villemure, M., and Taketo, T. (2008). The behavior of the X- and Y-chromosomes in the oocyte during meiotic prophase in the B6.Y^{TIR} sex-reversed mouse ovary. *Reproduction* 135, 241-252.

Amleh, A., Ledee, N., Saeed, J., and Taketo, T. (1996). Competence of oocytes from the B6.Y^{DOM} sex-reversed female mouse for maturation, fertilization, and embryonic development in vitro. *Dev. Biol.* 178, 263-275.

Amleh, A., Smith, L., Chen, H.-Y., and Taketo, T. (2000). Both nuclear and cytoplasmic components are defective in oocytes of the B6.Y^{TIR} sex-reversed female mouse. *Dev. Biol.* 219, 277-286.

Amleh, A. and Taketo, T. (1998). Live-borns from XX but not XY oocytes in the chimeric mouse ovary composed of B6.Y^{TIR} and XX cells. *Biol. Reprod.* 58, 574-582.

Anderson, E. and Albertini, D.F. (1976). Gap junctions between the oocyte and companion follicle cells in the mammalian ovary. *J. Cell Biol.* 71, 680-686.

Baarends, W.M., Wassenaar, E., van der Laan, R., Hoogerbrugge, J., Sleddens-Linkels, E., Hoejimakers, J.H.J., de Boer, P., and Grootegoed, J.A. (2005). Silencing of unpaired chromatin and histone H2A ubiquitination in mammalian meiosis. *Mol. Cell. Biol.* 25, 1041-1053.

Baker, T.G. (1963). A quantitative and cytological study of germ cells in human ovaries. *Proc. R. Soc. Lond.* B158, 417-433.

Behzadian, M.A., Tho, S.P.T., and McDonough, P.G. (1991). The presence of the testicular determining sequence, *SRY*, in 46, XY females with gonadal dysgenesis (Swyer syndrome). *Am. J. Obstet. Gynecol.* 165, 1887-1890.

Birgit, B., Julius, H., Carsten, R., Maryam, S., Gabriel, F., Victoria, K., Margareta, F., and Outi, H. (2009). Fertility preservation in girls with Turner syndrome: prognostic signs of the presence of ovarian follicles. *J. Clin. Endocrinol. Metab.* 94, 74-80.

Borum, K. (1961). Oogenesis in the mouse. A study of the meiotic prophase. *Exp. Cell Res.* 24, 495-507.

Brennan, J.B. and Capel, B. (2004). One tissue, two fates: Molecular genetics events that underlie testis versus ovary development. *Nature Rev. Genet.* 5, 509-521.

Bristol-Gould, S.K., Kreeger, P.K., Selkirk, C.G., Kilen, S.M., Cook, R.W., Kipp, J.L., Shea, L.D., Mayo, K.E., and Woodruff, T.K. (2006). Postnatal regulation of germ cells by activin: The establishment of the initial follicle pool. *Dev. Biol.* 298, 132-148.

Brook, J.D. (1983). X-chromosome segregation, maternal age and aneuploidy in the XO mouse. *Genet. Res. Camb.* 41, 85-95.

Brower, P.T. and Schultz, RM. (1982). Intracellular communication between granulosa cells and mouse oocytes: Existence and possible nutritional role during oocyte growth. *Dev. Biol.* 90, 144-153.

Buccione, R., Schroeder, A.C., and Eppig, J.J. (1990). Interactions between somatic cells and germ cells throughout mammalian oogenesis. *Biol. Reprod. 43*, 543-547.

Bullejos, M. and Koopman, P. (2005). Delayed *Sry* and *Sox9* expression in developing mouse gonads underlies B6-Y^{DOM} sex reversal. *Dev. Biol. 278*, 473-481.

Burgoyne, P.S. and Baker, T.G. (1981). Oocytes depletion in XO mice and their XX sibs from 12 to 200 days post partum. *J. Reprod. Fert. 61*, 207-212.

Burgoyne, P.S. and Baker, T.G. (1985). Perinatal oocyte loss in XO mice and its implications for the aetiology of gonadal dysgenesis in XO women. *J. Reprod. Fert. 75*, 633-645.

Burgoyne, P.S. and Biggers, J.D. (1976). The consequences of X-dosage deficiency in the germ line: impaired development in vitro of preimplantation embryos from XO mice. *Dev. Biol.* 51, 109-117.

Burgoyne, P.S. and Evans, E.P. (2000). A high frequency of XO offspring from $X^{Paf}Y*$ male mice: evidence that the *Paf* mutation involves an inversion spanning the X PAR boundary. *Cytogenet. Cell Genet.* 91, 57-61.

Burgoyne, P.S., Mahadevaiah, S.K., and Turner, J.M.A. (2009). The consequences of asynapsis for mammalian meiosis. *Nature Rev. Genet.* 10, 207-216.

Burgoyne, P.S. and Rastan, S. (1991). Prenatal selection in XO mice. *Nature* 353, 709.

Burgoyne, P.S., Tam, P.P.L., and Evans, E.P. (1983). Retarded development of XO conceptuses during early pregnancy in the mouse. *J. Reprod. Fert.* 68, 387-393.

Cameron, F.J. and Sinclair, A.H. (1997). Mutations in *SRY* and *SOX9*: testis-determining genes. *Hum. Mutation* 9, 388-395.

Capel, B., Rasberry, C., Dyson, J., Bishop, C.E., Simpson, E., Vivian, N., Lovell-Badge, R., Rastan, S., and Cattanach, B.M. (1993). Deletion of Y chromosome sequences located outside the testis determining region can cause XY female sex reversal. *Nature Genet.* 5, 301-307.

Cattanach, B.M. (1962). XO mice. *Genet. Res. Camb.* 3, 487-490.

Chuva De Sousa Lopes, S.M., Hayashi, K., Shovlin, T.C., Mifsud, W., Surani, M.A., and McLaren, A. (2008). X chromosome activity in mouse XX primordial germ cells. *PLos Genet.* 3, e30.

Cotinot, C., Pailhoux, E., Jaubert, F., and Fellous, M. (2002). Molecular genetics of sex determination. *Sem. Reprod. Med.* 20, 157-167.

Coward, P., Nagai, K., Chen, D., Thomas, H.D., Nagamine, C.M., and Lau, Y.C. (1994). Polymorphism of a CAG trinucleotide repeat within *Sry* correlates with B6.Y^{DOM} sex reversal. *Nature Genet.* 6, 245-250.

Davies, W., Isles, A., Smith, R., Karunadasa, D., Burrmann, D., Humby, T., Ojarikre, O., Biggin, C., Skuse, D., Burgoyne, P., and Wilkinson, L. (2005). *Xlr3b* is a new imprinted candidate for X-linked parent-of-origin effects on cognitive function in mice. *Nature Genet.* 37, 625-629.

Deckers, J.F.M. and Van der Kroon, P.H.W. (1981). Some characteristics of the XO mouse (*Mus musculus L.*) I. Vitality: Growth and metabolism. *Genetica* 55, 179-185.

Dubin, R.A., Coward, P., Lau, Y.-F.C., and Oster, H. (1995). Functional comparison of the *Mus musculus molessinus* and *Mus musculus domesticus Sry* genes. *Mol. Endocrinol.* 9, 1645-1654.

Dumic, M., Lin-Su, K., Leibel, N.I., Ciglar, S., Vinci, G., Lasan, R., Nimkarn, S., Wilson, J.D., McElreavey, K., and New, M.I. (2008). Report of fertility in a woman with a predominantly 46,XY karyotype in a family with multiple disorders of sexual development. *J. Clin. Endocrinol. Metab.* 93, 182-189.

Eicher, E.M., Shown, E.P., and Washburn, L.L. (1995). Sex reversal in C57BL/6J-Y^{POS} mice corrected by a *Sry* transgene. *Phil. Trans. R. Soc. Lond.* B350, 263-269.

Eicher, E.M. and Washburn, L.L. (1986). Genetic control of primary sex determination in mice. *Ann. Rev. Genet.* 20, 327-360.

Eicher, E.M., Washburn, L.L., Whitney, J.B.I., and Morrow, K.E. (1982). *Mus poshiavinus* Y chromosome in the C57BL/6J murine genome causes sex reversal. *Science* 217, 535-537.

Eppig, J.J. (2005). Mouse oocytes control metabolic co-operativity between oocytes and cumulus cells. *Reprod. Fert. Dev.* 17, 1-2.

Espinosa, M.B. and Vitullo, A.D. (1996). Offspring sex-ratio and reproductive performance in heterogametic females of the South American field mouse *Akodon azarae*. Reproduction in heterogametic *Akodon azarae* females. *Hereditas* 124, 57-62.

Evans, E.P. and Phillips, R.J.S. (1975). Inversion heterozygosity and the origin of XO daughters of *Bpa*/+ female mice. *Nature* 256, 40-41.

Fisher, E.M.C., Beer-Romero, P., Brown, L.G., Ridley, A., McNeil, J.A., Lawrence, J.B., Willard, H.F., Bieber, F.R., and Page, D.C. (1990). Homologous ribosomal protein genes on the human X and Y chromosomes: Escape from X inactivation and possible implications for Turner syndrome. *Cell* 63, 1205-1218.

Foster, J.W., Dominguez-Steglich, M.A., Guioli, S., Kwok, C., Weller, P.A., Stevanovic, M., Weissenbach, J., Monsour, S., Young, I.D., Goodfellow, P.N., Brook, J.D., and Schafer, A.J. (1994). Campomelic dysplasia and autosomal sex reversal caused by mutations in an SRY-related gene. *Nature* 372, 525-530.

Frydman, R., Parneix, I., Fries, N., Testart, J., Raymond, J.-P., and Bouchard, P. (1988). Pregnancy in a 46, XY patient. *Fert. Steril.* 50, 813-814.

Hall, H., Hunt, P., and Hassold, T. (2006). Meiosis and sex chromosome aneuploidy: how meiotic errors cause aneuploidy; how aneuploidy causes meiotic errors. *Curr. Op. Genet. Dev.* 16, 323-329.

Harley, V.R., Jackson, D.I., Hextall, P.J., Hawkins, J.R., Berkovitz, G.D., Sockanathan, S., Lovell-Badge, R., and Goodfellow, P.N. (1992). DNA binding activity of recombinant SRY from normal males and XY females. *Science* 255, 453-456.

Harley, V.R., Layfield, S., Mitchel, C.L., Forwood, J.K., John, A.P., Briggs, L.J., McDowall, S.G., and Jans, D.A. (2003). Defective importin β recognition and nuclear import of the sex-determining factor SRY are associated with XY sex-reversing mutations. *Proc. Natl. Acad. Sci. USA* 100, 7045-7050.

Hoekstra, H.E. (2003). Unequal transmission of mitochondrial haplotypes in natural populations of field mice with XY females (genus *Akodon*). *Am. Nat.* 161, 29-39.

Hoekstra, H.E. and Hoekstra, J.M. (2001). An unusual sex-determination system in south American field mice (genus *AKODON*): the role of mutation, selection, and meiotic drive in maintaining XY females. *Evolution* 55, 190-197.

Hreinsson, J.G., Otala, M., Fridström, M., Borgström, B., Rasmussen, C., Lundqvist, M., Tuuri, T., Simberg, N., Mikkola, M., Dunkel. L., and Hovatta, O. (2002). Follicles are found in the ovaries of adolescent girls with Turner's syndrome. *J. Clin. Endocrinol. Metab.* 87, 3618-3623.

Hunt, P.A. (1991). Survival of XO mouse fetuses: effect of parental origin of the X chromosome or uterin environment? *Development* 111, 1137-1141.

Ishikawa, H., Rattigan, A., Fundale, R., and Burgoyne, P.S. (2003). Effects of sex chromosome dosage on placental size in mice. *Biol. Reprod.* 69, 483-488.

Jacobs, P., Dalton, P., James, R., Mosse, K., Power, M., Rovinson, D., and Skuse, D. (1997). Turner syndrome: a cytogenetic and molecular study. *Ann. Hum. Genet.* 61, 471-483.

Jamieson, R.V., Tan, S.-S., and Tam, P.P.L. (1998). Retarded postimplantation development of XO mouse embryos: impact of the parental origin of the monosomic X chromosome. *Dev. Biol.* 201, 13-25.

Kapalanga, J. and Blecher, S.R. (1990). Effect of the X-linked gene *Tabby* (*Ta*) on eyelid opening and incisor eruption in neonatal mice is opposite to that of epidermal growth factor. *Development* 108, 349-355.

Kashimada, K. and Koopman, P. (2010). *Sry*: The master switch in mammalian sex determination. *Development* 137, 3921-3930.

Kaufman, M.H. (1972). Non-random segregation during mammalian oogenesis. *Nature* 238, 465-466.

Kaur, G., Delluc-Clavieres, A., Poon, I.K.H., Forwood, J.K., Glover, D.J., and Jans, D.A. (2010). Calmodulin-dependent nuclear import of HMG-box family nuclear factors: Importance of the role of SRY in sex reversal. *Biochem. J.* 430, 39-48.

Kim, Y., Kobayashi, A., Sekido, R., DiNapoli, L., Brennan, J., Chaboissier, M.-C., Poulat, F., Behringer, R.R., Lovell-Badge, R., and Capel, B. (2006). Fgf9 and Wnt4 act as antagonistic signals to regulate mammalian sex determination. *PLos Biol.* 4, e187

Koehler, K.E., Millie, E.A., Cherry, J.P., Burgoyne, P.S., Evens, E.P., Hunt, P.A., and Hassold, T.J. (2002). Sex-specific differences in meiotic chromosome segregation revealed by dicentric bridge resolution in mice. *Genetics* 162, 1367-1379.

Koopman, P., Gubbary, J., Vivian, N., Goodfellow, P., and Lovell-Badge, R. (1991). Male development of chromosomally female mice transgenic for *Sry*. *Nature* 351, 117-121.

Kouznetsova, A., Wang, H., Bellani, M., Camerini-Otero, R.D., Jessberger, R., and Hoog, C. (2009). BRCA1-mediated chromatin silencing is limited to oocytes with a small number of asynapsed chromosomes. *J. Cell Sci.* 122, 2446-2452.

Kwok, C., Goodfellow, P.N., and Hawkins, J.R. (1996). Evidence to exclude *SOX9* as a candidate gene for XY sex reversal without skeltal malformation. *J. Med. Genet.* 33, 800-801.

Lane, P.W. and Davisson, M.T. (1990). *Patchy Fur* (*Paf*), a semidominant X-linked gene associated with a high level of X-Y nondisjunction in male mice. *J. Heredity* 81, 43-50.

Lau, Y.-F.C. (1999). Sex chromosome genetics '99. Gonadoblastoma, testicular and prostate cancers, and the *TSPY* gene. *Am. J. Hum. Genet.* 64, 921-927.

Lavery, R., Lardenois, A., Ranc-Jianmotamedi, F., Pauper, E., Gregoire, E.P., Vigier, C., Moreilhon, C., Primig, M., and Chaboissier, M.-C. (2011). XY *Sox9* embryonic loss-of-function mouse mutants show complete sex reversal and produce partially fertile XY oocytes. *Dev. Biol.* 354, 111-122.)

Lawson, K.A., Dunn, N.R., Roelen, B.A.J., Zeinstra, L.M., Davis, A.M., Wright, C.V.E., Korving, J.P.W.F.M., and Hogan, B.L.M. (1999). Bmp4 is required for the generation of primordial germ cells in the mouse embryos. *Genes Dev.* 13, 424-436.

Lee, C.-H. and Taketo, T. (1994). Normal onset, but prolonged expression, of *Sry* gene in the B6.Y^{DOM} sex-reversed mouse gonad. *Dev. Biol.* 165, 442-452.

Lee, C.-H. and Taketo, T. (2001). Low levels of *Sry* transcripts cannot be the sole cause of B6.Y^{TIR} sex reversal. *Genesis* 30, 7-11.

Lim, H.N., Freestone, S.H., Romero, D., Kwok, C., Hughes, I.A., and Hawkins, J.R. (1998). Candidate genes in complete and partial XY sex reversal: Mutation analysis of *SRY*, SRY-related genes and *FTZ-F1*. *Mol. Cell. Endocrinol.* 140, 51-58.

Lovell-Badge, R. and Robertson, E. (1990). XY female mice resulting from a heritable mutation in the primary testis-determining gene, *Tdy*. *Development* 109, 635-646.

Luthardt, F.W. (1976). Cytogenetic analysis of oocytes and early preimplantation embryos from XO mice. *Dev. Biol.* 54, 73-81.

Lyon, M.F. and Hawker, S.G. (1973). Reproductive lifespan in irradiated and unirradiated chromosomally XO mice. *Genet. Res. Camb.* 21, 185-194.

Maatouk, D.M., DiNapoli, L., Alvers, A., Parker, K.L., Taketo, M.M., and Capel, B. (2008). Stabilization of β-catenin in XY gonads causes male-to-female sex-reversal. *Hum. Mol. Genet.* 17, 2949-2955.

MacDonald, M., Hassold, T., Harvey, J., Wang, L.H., Morton, N.E., and Jacobs, P. (1994). The origin of 47,XXY and 47,XXX aneuploidy: heterogeneous mechanisms and role of aberrant recombination. *Hum. Mol. Genet.* 3, 1365-1371.

Magee, A.C. and Hughes, A.E. (1998). Segregation distortion in myotonic dystrophy. *J. Med. Genet.* 35, 1045-1046.

Mahadevaiah, S.K., Bourc'his, D., de Rooij, D.G., Bestor, T.H., Turner, J.M.A., and Burgoyne, P.S. (2008). Extensive meiotic asynapsis in mice antagonises meiotic silencing of unsynapsed chromatin and consequently disrupts meiotic sex chromosome inactivation. *J. Cell Biol.* 182, 263-276.

Mahadevaiah, S.K., Lovell-Badge, R., and Burgoyne, P.S. (1993). *Tdy*-negative XY, XXY and XYY female mice: breeding data and synaptonemal complex analysis. *J. Reprod. Fert.* 97, 151-160.

Manuel, M., Katayama, K.P., and Jones, H.W. (1976). The age of occurrence of gonadal tumors in intersex patients with a Y chromosome. *Am. J. Obstet. Gynecol.* 124, 293-299.

Marmolejo-Valencia, A., Nishioka, Y., Moreno-Mendoza, N., and Merchant-Larios, H. (1999). Fertility of Y^{TIR}.B6 sex-reversal females with XX orthotopic ovarian transplants. *Biol. Reprod.* 61, 1426-1430.

May, K.M., Jacobs, P.A., Lee, M., Ratcliffe, S., Robinson, A., Neilsen, J., and Hassold, T.J. (1990). The parental origin of the extra X chromosome in 47,XXX females. *Am. J. Hum. Genet.* 46, 754-761.

Merchant-Larios, H., Clarke, H.J., and Taketo, T. (1994). Developmental arrest of fertilized eggs from the B6.Y^{DOM} sex-reversed female mouse. *Dev. Genet.* 15, 435-442.

Meyer, J., Südbeck, P., Held, M., Wagner, T., Schmitz, M.L., Bricarelli, F.D., Eggermont, E., Friedrich, U., Haas, O.A., Kobelt, A., Leroy, J.G., Van Maldergem, L., Michel, E., Mitulla, B., Pfeiffer, R.A., Schinzel, A., Schmidt, H., and Scherer, G. (1997). Mutational analysis of the *SOX9* gene in campomelic dysplasia and autosomal sex reversal: lack of genotype/phenotype correlations. *Hum. Mol. Genet.* 6, 91-98.

Modi, D.N., Sane, S., and Bhartiya, D. (2003). Accelerated germ cell apoptosis in sex chromosome aneuploid fetal human gonads. *Mol. Hum. Reprod.* 9, 219-225.

Molyneaux, K.A., Stallock, J., Schaible, K., and Wylie, C. (2001). Time-lapse analysis of living mouse germ cell migration. *Dev. Biol.* 240, 488-498.

Monk, M. and McLaren, A. (1981). X-chromosome activity in foetal germ cells of the mouse. *J. Embryol. exp. Morph.* 63, 75-84.

Moreno-Mendoza, N., Torres-Maldonado, L., Chimal-Monroy, J., Harley, V., and Merchant-Larios, H. (2004). Disturbed expression of Sox9 in pre-Sertoli cells underlines sex-reversal in mice, B6.Y^{tir-1}. *Biol. Reprod.* 70, 114-122.

Mullen, R.J. and Whitten, W.K. (1971). Relationship of genotype and degree of chimerism in coat color to sex ratios and gametogenesis in chimeric mice. *J. Exp. Zool.* 178, 165-176.

Nagamine, C.M., Morohashi, K., Carlisle, C., and Chang, D.K. (1999). Sex reversal caused by *Mus musclus domesticus* Y chromosomes linked to variant expression of the testis-determining gene *Sry*. *Dev. Biol.* 216, 182-194.

Nagamine, C.M., Taketo, T., and Koo, G.C. (1987a). Morphological development of the mouse gonad in *tda-1* XY sex reversal. *Differentiation* 33, 214-222.

Nagamine, C.M., Taketo, T., and Koo, G.C. (1987b). Studies on the genetics of *tda-1* XY sex reversal in the mouse. *Differentiation* 33, 223-231.

Nguyen, D.K. and Disteche, C.M. (2006). Dosage compensation of the active X chromosome in mammals. *Nature Genet.* 38, 47-53.

Nielsen, J. and Wohlert, M. (1991). Chromosome abnormalities found among 34910 newborn children: Results from a 13-year incidence study in Arhus, Denmark. *Hum. Genet.* 87, 81-83.

Obata, Y., Villemure, M., Kono, T., and Taketo, T. (2008). Transmission of Y chromosomes from XY female mice was made possible by the replacement of cytoplasm during oocyte maturation. *Proc. Natl. Acad. Sci. USA* 105, 13918-13923.

Omoe, K. and Endo, A. (1993). Growth and development of 39,X mouse embryos at mid-gestation. *Cytogenet. Cell Genet.* 63, 50-53.

Ottolenghi, C., Omari, S., Garcia-Ortiz, J.E., Uda, M., Crisponi, L., Forabosco, A., Pilia, G., and Schlessinger, D. (2005). Foxl2 is required for commitment to ovary differentiation. *Hum. Mol. Genet.* 14, 2053-2062.

Park, E.-H. and Taketo, T. (2003). Onset and progress of meiotic prophase in the oocytes in the B6.Y^{TIR} sex-reversed mouse ovary. *Biol. Reprod.* 69, 1879-1889.

Park, S., Zeidan, K.T., Shin, J.S., and Taketo, T. (2011). SRY upregulation of SOX9 is inefficient and delayed, allowing ovarian differentiation, in the B6.Y^{TIR} gonad. *Differentiation* 82, 18-27.

Park, S.Y. and Jameson, J.L. (2005). Minireview: transcriptional regulation of gonadal development and differentiation. *Endocrinology* 146, 1035-1042.

Park, S.Y., Lee, E.-J., Emge, D., Jahn, C.L., and Jameson, J.L. (2008). A phenotypic spectrum of sexual development in *Dax1* (*Nr0b1*)-deficient mice: consequence of the C57BL/6J strain on sex determination. *Biol. Reprod.* 79, 1038-1045.

Phillips, R.J.S., Hawker, S.G., and Moseley, H.J. (1973). Bare-patches, a new sex-linked gene in the mouse, associated with a high production of XO females. I. A preliminary report of breeding experiments. *Genet. Res. Camb.* 22, 91-99.

Prothero, K.E., Stahl, J.M., and Carrel, L. (2009). Dosage compensation and gene expression on the mammalian X chromosome: one plus one does not always equal two. *Chromosome Res.* 17, 637-648.

Raefski, A.S. and O'Neill, M.J. (2005). Identification of a cluster of X-linked imprinted genes in mice. *Nature Genet.* 37, 620-624.

Russel, W.L., Russell, L.B., and Gower, J.S. (1959). Exceptional inheritance of a sex-linked gene in the mouse explained on the basis that the X/O sex-chromosome constitution is female. *Proc. Natl. Acad. Sci. USA* 45, 554-560.

Sakurada, K., Omoe, K., and Endo, A. (1994). Increased incidence of unpartnered single chromatids in metaphase II oocytes in 39,X(XO) mice. *Experientia* 50, 502-505.

Schartl, M. (2004). Sex chromosome evolution in non-mammalian vertebrates. *Curr. Op. Genet. Dev.* 14, 634-641.

Sekido, R. and Lovell-Badge, R. (2008). Sex determination and SRY: down to a wink and a nudge? *Trends Genet.* 25, 19-29.

Shao, C. and Takagi, N. (1990). An extra maternally derived X chromosome is deleterious to early mouse development. *Development* 110, 969-975.

Sim, H., Rimmer, K., Kelly, S., Ludbrook, L.M., Clayton, A.H.A., and Harley, V.R. (2005). Defective calmodulin-mediated nuclear transport of the sex-determining region of the Y chromosome (SRY) in XY sex reversal. *Mol. Endocrinol.* 19, 1884-1892.

Sinclair, A.H., Berta, P., Palmer, M.S., Hawkins, J.R., Griffiths, B.L., Smith, M.J., Foster, J.W., Frischauf, A.-M., Lovell-Badge, R., and Goodfellow, P.N. (1990). A gene from the human sex-determining region encodes a protein with homology to a conserved DNA-binding motif. *Nature* 346, 240-244.

Singh, L., Matsukuma, S., and Jones, K.W. (1987). Testis development in a mouse with 10 % of XY cells. *Dev. Biol.* 122, 287-290.

Speed, R.M. (1982). Meiosis in the foetal mouse ovary. I. An analysis at the light microscope level using surface-spreading. *Chromosoma* (Berl) 85, 427-437.

Speed, R.M. (1986). Oocyte development in XO foetuses of man and mouse: The possible role of heterologous X-chromosome pairing in germ cell survival. *Chromosoma* (Berl.) 94, 115-124.

Stratakis, C.A. and Rennert, O.M. (2005). Turner syndrome an update. *Endocrinologists* 15, 27-36.

Sugimoto, M.A.K.2.P.G.3.7.pp.pp. (2007). X chromosome reactivation initiates in nascent primordial germ cells in mice. *PLoS Genet.* 3, e116.

Sugiura, K. and Eppig, J.J. (2005). Society for Reproductive Biology founders'lecture 2005. Control of metabolic cooperativity between oocytes and their companion granulosa cells by mouse oocytes. *Reprod. Fert. Dev.* 17, 667-674.

Taketo-Hosotani, T., Nishioka, Y., Nagamine, C., Villalpando, I., and Merchant-Larios, H. (1989). Development and fertility of ovaries in the B6.Y^{DOM} sex-reversed female mouse. *Development* 197, 95-105.

Taketo, T., Lee, C.-H., Zhang, J., Li, Y., Lee, C.-Y.G., and Lau, Y.-F.C. (2005). Expression of SRY proteins in both normal and sex-reversed XY fetal mouse gonads. *Dev. Dyn.* 233, 612-622.

Tam, P.P.L. and Zhou, S.X. (1996). The allocation of epiblast cells to ectodermal and germ-line lineages is influenced by the position of the cells in the gastrulating mouse embryo. *Dev. Biol.* 178, 124-132.

Tarani, L., Lampariello, S., Raguso, G., Colloridi, F., Pucarelli, I., Pasquino, A.M., and Bruni, L.A. (1998). Pregnancy in patients with Turner's syndrome: Six new cases and review of literature. *Gynecol. Endocrinol.* 12, 83-87.

Thornhill, A.R. and Burgoyne, P.S. (1993). A paternally imprinted X chromosome retards the development of the early mouse embryo. *Development* 118, 171-174.

Tulic, I., Tulic, L., and Micic, J. (2011). Pregnancy in patient with Swyer syndrome. *Fert. Steril.* 95, 1789.

Turner, J.M.A., Mahadevaiah, S.K., Fernandes-Capetillo, O., Nussenzweig, A., Xu, X., Deng, C.-X., and Burgoyne, P.S. (2005). Silencing of unsynapsed meiotic chromosomes in the mouse. *Nature Genet.* 37, 41-47.

Uehara, S., Funato, T., Yaegashi, N., Suziki, H., Sato, J., Sasaki, T., and Yajima, A. (1999). SRY mutation and tumor formation on the gonads of XY pure gonadal dysgenesis patients. *Cancer Genet. Cytogenet.* 113, 78-84.

Vaiman, D. and Pailhoux, E. (2000). Mammalian sex reversal and intersexuality. *Trends Genet.* 16, 488-494.

Villalpando, I., Nishioka, Y., and Taketo, T. (1993). Endocrine differentiation of the XY sex-reversed mouse ovary during postnatal development. *J. Steroid Biochem. Mol. Biol.* 45, 265-273.

Villemure, M., Chen, H.-Y., Kurokawa, M., Fissore, R.A., and Taketo, T. (2007). The presence of X- and Y-chromosomes in oocytes leads to impairment in the progression of the second meiotic division. *Dev. Biol.* 301, 1-13.

Wagner, T., Wirth, J., Meyer, J., Zabel, B., Held, M., Zimmer, J., Pasantes, J., Bricarelli, F.D., Keutel, J., Hustert, E., Wolf, U., Tommerup, N., Schempp, W., and Scherer, G. (1994). Autosomal sex reversal and Campomelic dysplasia are caused by mutations in and around the SRY-related gene *SOX9*. *Cell* 79, 1111-1120.

Welshons, W.J. and Russell, L.B. (1959). The Y chromosome as the bearer of male determining factors in the mouse. *Proc. Natl. Acad. Sci. USA* 45, 560-566.

Wilhelm, D., Palmer, S., and Koopman, P. (2007). Sex determination and gonadal development in mammals. *Physiol. Rev.* 87, 1-28.

Wong, J., Luckers, L., Okawara, Y., Pelletier, R.-M., and Taketo, T. (2000). Follicular development and atresia in the B6.Y^{TIR} sex-reversed mouse ovary. *Biol. Reprod.* 63, 756-762.

Xu, B.-Z., Obata, Y., Cao, F., and Taketo, T. (2012). The presence of the Y-chromosome, not the absence of the second X-chromosome, alters the mRNAs stored in the fully grown XY mouse oocyte. *PLos One* 7, e40481.

Yang, F., Babak, T., Shendure, J., and Disteche, C.M. (2010). Global survey of escape from X inactivation by RNA-sequencing in mouse. *Genome Res.* 20, 614-622.

Yang, H., Shi, L., Wang, B.-A., Liang, D., Zhong, C., Liu, W., Nie, Y., Liu, J., Zhao, J., Gao, X., Li, D., Xu, G.-L., and Li, J. (2012). Generation of genetically modified mice by oocyte injection of androgenetic haploid embryonic stem cells. *Cell* 605-617.

In: Sex Chromosomes: New Research
Editors: M. D'Aquino and V. Stallone

ISBN: 978-1-62417-143-7
© 2013 Nova Science Publishers, Inc.

Chapter III

The Fate of the Y Chromosome

Asato Kuroiwa[*]

Laboratory of Animal Cytogenetics, Department of Biological Sciences,
Faculty of Science, Hokkaido University, Japan

Abstract

The mammalian X and Y chromosomes were originally a homologous pair of chromosomes. The accumulation of deleterious mutations and the subsequent inactivation and loss of Y-linked genes could have led to the genetic degeneration of the Y chromosome over evolutionary time, approximately 300 million years (Myr). In modern humans, only approximately 45 Y-linked genes remain. Most of these have acquired functions that are essential for maleness, for example, sex determination or spermatogenesis. It has been proposed that the loss of human Y-linked genes is inexorable and might lead to the extinction of the entire species because of the active role that this chromosome plays in male function. The contrary opinion suggests that the remaining Y-linked genes are strictly conserved through purifying selection. Recent comparative genomic analysis among the Y-chromosome sequences of primates, human, chimpanzee, and rhesus macaque, showed a high level of conservation of human Y-linked genes, at least over the past 25 Myr of the human lineage. However, rodents include very interesting species in which complete loss of the Y chromosome has occurred. Two species of

---

[*] Address: North10, West8, Kita-ku, Sapporo, Japan, 060-0810. Tell: +81-11-706-2752; FAX: +81-11-706-2619. E-mail: asatok@sci.hokudai.ac.jp.

Ryukyu spiny rat and one species of mole vole have an XO/XO sex chromosome constitution due to absence of the Y chromosome. Furthermore, in these species, a key mammalian sex-determining gene, *SRY*, was also lost upon disappearance of the Y chromosome. These XO species show us that loss of the Y chromosome would not lead to the extinction of humans, and there are several processes of Y evolution in our future.

Introduction

The sex of mammals is genetically determined by the inheritance of sex chromosomes at the time of fertilization. If the constitution of the sex chromosomes is XX, the fertilized egg develops into a female. If the constitution is XY, it becomes a male. The mammalian X chromosome is relatively large. It comprises approximately 5% of the haploid genome, and in general the size of the X chromosome is conserved in mammals, with a few exceptions [1]. In contrast, the mammalian Y chromosome is extremely small and contains very few genes. This small number of genes has acquired male-specific functions, for example, in sex determination and spermatogenesis, which means that they are essential for maleness in mammals. Recently, two different hypotheses regarding the future fate of the Y chromosome have been proposed: (i) the Y chromosome will disappear as a consequence of the complete loss of all its genes, or (ii) the Y chromosome will survive because the Y-linked genes are necessary for males.

This chapter describes the degeneration process that the human Y chromosome has undergone in the past, as well as features of the human Y-linked genes. In addition, it presents recent findings from comparative genomic analysis among primate Y chromosomes and a series of studies on mammals in which the Y chromosome is actually absent.

The Degeneration Process of the Y Chromosome

The mammalian X and Y chromosomes have co-evolved from an ordinary pair of autosomes in the common ancestor of mammals, which first appeared approximately 300 million years (Myr) ago [2-4]. During the course of evolution, X-Y crossing over was suppressed in five different chromosome regions at five different times, with each suppression probably resulting from an inversion in the Y chromosome (Figure 1) [3, 4]. Each inversion enlarged the portion of the X and Y chromosomes that did not recombine during male meiosis. This led to the accumulation of deleterious mutations in Y-linked genes caused by the reduced efficacy of purifying selection in non-recombining regions [5]. The subsequent inactivation and loss of Y-linked genes lead to the genetic degeneration of the Y chromosome.

Comparison of the present-day X and Y chromosomes enables the identification of the five evolutionary "strata" in the male-specific region of the Y chromosome (MSY) and the X chromosome (Figure 1) [3, 4]. Their distinctive degrees of X-Y differentiation indicate the evolutionary ages of the strata. The oldest stratum (stratum 1) dates back more than 240 Myr and is the most highly differentiated between the X and Y chromosomes [3], whereas the youngest stratum (stratum 5) originated only 30 Myr ago and displays the highest X-Y nucleotide sequence similarity within the MSY [4].

The prototype of the human Y chromosome contained more than 1,000 genes. However, all but approximately 45 have been inactivated or lost. This gives an inactivation rate of 3.3 genes per Myr, which suggests that the Y chromosome might last only another 14 Myr [7].

Possible trajectories for the degeneration of the human Y chromosome from 300 Myr ago up to the present time have been proposed (Figure 2) [7]: (i) the rate of loss of active genes was constant, (ii) the number of active genes showed an exponential decline, (iii) a target size of gene-loss that initially increased and then decreased or (iv) an exponential decline that was slowed down in its final stages by positive selection. Furthermore, it has been proposed that the loss of human Y-linked genes is inexorable and might lead to the extinction of the entire species because of the vital role that this chromosome plays in male function [8] (e.g., male sex determination, testis development, and spermatogenesis; see next section).

This hypothesis is of great interest. Could the degeneration of the Y chromosome continue until nothing remains? Will the gene-poor mammalian Y chromosome disappear in the future?

The Y-Linked Genes – Sex Determination and Spermatogenesis

The most well-known Y-linked gene is *SRY* (sex-determining region Y). The *SRY* gene is a molecular switch for sex determination in placental mammals, and acts as a trigger for testis development in the undifferentiated gonads of an embryo.

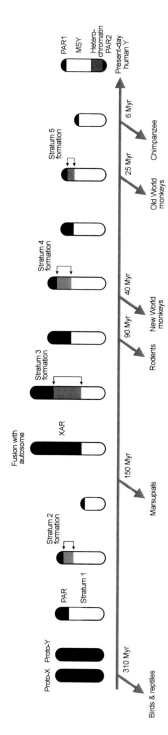

Figure 1. The evolution process and strata formation of the human Y chromosome (Hughes and Rozen, 2012 [6] was modified). The mammalian X and Y chromosomes have co-evolved from an ordinary pair of autosomes in the common ancestor of mammals, which first appeared 310 million years (Myr) ago. During the course of evolution, the five evolutionary "strata" have appeared in the male-specific region of the Y chromosome (MSY) resulting from mainly five inversions at five different times. X-Y recombining regions are shown in black. The enlarged portion of the X and Y chromosomes that did not recombine during male meiosis caused by inversion are shown in gray. Arrows indicate inversions. MSYs that have differentiated from the X chromosome are shown in white. The major heterochromatic region on the present-day human Y chromosome is shown in dark gray. XAR (X-added region) indicates that the region in which an autosome was added. PAR1 and PAR2 indicate short-arm pseudoautosomal region and long-arm pseudoautosomal resion, respectively.

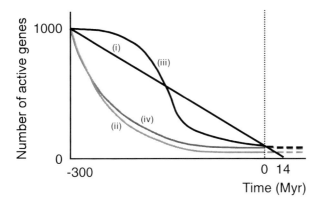

Figure 2. Possible trajectories for the degeneration of the human Y chromosome from 300 Myr ago up to the present time (Graves 2006 [7] was modified). The rate of loss of active genes was constant (i), the number of active genes showed an exponential decline (ii), a target size of gene-loss that initially increased and then decreased (iii) or an exponential decline that was slowed down in its final stages by positive selection (iv).

It was known that the majority of human XX males possess a Y-derived DNA sequence owing to part of the Y-chromosome region that includes the gene for TDF (testis-determining factor) being transferred to the X chromosome by aberrant X-Y interchange during meiosis [9, 10]. An analysis of the Y-derived 35-kb region of XX males was undertaken, which resulted in the identification of an open reading frame (ORF) for *SRY* [11]. In addition, mutations in *SRY* were identified in XY females, which showed that *SRY* function is normally required for testis development [12, 13]. Furthermore, a homologous gene of mouse was found [14], and XX transgenic mice of *Sry* showed the male phenotype: testes and male external genitalia [15]. These reports demonstrated that only one gene on the Y chromosome is necessary to initiate the cascade of male development, and that *SRY/Sry* encodes the testis-determining factor.

SRY has been shown to function as a transcription factor that activates *Sox9* expression by binding to the *Sox9* (SRY-box containing gene 9) enhancer together with the NR5A1 protein (nuclear receptor subfamily 5, group A, member 1, also known as AD4BP/SF1) in the undifferentiated gonads of XY embryos [16]. The DNA-binding domain named the HMG box is very important for this DNA-binding function of *SRY/Sry* because even one amino acid substitution in the HMG box can produce a sex reversal, namely, an XY female [17]. Further study revealed that the sex of most placental species is determined by the *SRY* gene on the Y chromosome. In addition, the amino acid sequence of the HMG box is highly conserved among placental species, whereas the rate of evolutionary change in the region outside the HMG box is very high [18].

Many other testis-specific genes were identified that were suspected of functioning in spermatogenesis. However, several other Y-linked genes were found to be expressed ubiquitously and had no obvious male-specific function. At the turn of century, the human Y-linked genes were classified into three groups on the basis of their expression profiles and homology to their X homologues [19]. Class 1 genes have a single copy, are expressed widely in the body, and have functions similar to those of their X homologues. Class 2 genes have multiple copies, are expressed only in the testis, and lack an active X homologue. Class 3 genes could not be as clearly defined as class 1 or 2 genes. *SRY* is categorized into class 3.

A single copy of *SRY* is expressed specifically in the embryonic undifferentiated gonads as the master trigger of testis development (as mentioned above) and it has an active X homologue, *SOX3* (SRY-box 3). Another class 3 gene is *AMELY* (amelogenin, Y-linked), which has an active X homologue, *AMELX* (amelogenin, X-linked). *AMELY* and *AMELX* are expressed only in developing tooth buds [20]. *RBMY1A1* (RNA-binding motif protein, Y-linked, family 1, member A1) also has features of both class 1 and class 2 genes. Similarly to class 1 genes, it has an active X homologue, *RBMX* (RNA-binding motif protein, X-linked). Similarly to class 2 genes, it is expressed from multiple copies, but only in the testes [21, 22].

Comparison of Human and Primate Y Chromosomes

From 2005 to 2010, two main research groups focused on sequencing and analyzing the Y-chromosome sequences of our closest living relative, the chimpanzee (*Pan troglodytes*, Hominidae, Primates) [23-25]. By comparing the Y-chromosome sequences of chimpanzee and human, substantial differences were identified in terms of sequence structure and gene content. These differences have accumulated independently during the past 6 Myr since the divergence of their lineages. In the human lineage, Y-linked genes were conserved through purifying selection. In contrast, gene decay in the chimpanzee lineage might have been a consequence of positive selection that was focused elsewhere on the Y chromosome [23-25]. Specifically, the human MSY has not lost any genes since the human–chimpanzee lineages diverged approximately 6 Myr ago. The accelerated rate of evolution of the Y chromosome, together with recent changes in the population size of the great apes and changes in human society related to reproductive behavior, might have had additional effects on the composition of the Y chromosomes of these two species. Sperm competition was suggested as a major factor that could have caused rapid and radical changes in the lineage of modern chimpanzees, in which several males mate with the same female at each oestrus. The heightened sperm competition in the chimpanzee lineage, together with positive selection and hitchhiking effects, might account for the greater amplification of MSY sequences in chimpanzees than in humans, and extensive gene loss compared with little or none in the human MSY.

The most recent evolutionary stratum among the five strata in the human Y chromosome (stratum 5) was established 30 Myr ago [4], which was 5 Myr before the human and Old World monkey lineages diverged (Figure 1). Consequently, comparison of this stratum of the human MSY and that of Old World monkeys should be very useful to determine the genes that were lost during the last 25 Myr. Dr. Jennifer F. Hughes and colleagues reported the Y-chromosome sequence of the rhesus macaque (*Macaca mulatta*, Cercopithecidae, Primates) in 2012 [26], and compared its MSY with that of humans [5]. The results are of great interest: the numbers and types of genes in rhesus macaques and humans have been largely maintained, despite the long time since the divergence of these lineages, namely 25 Myr. In the four oldest strata (strata 1–4), which were established 300–40 Myr ago, the compositions of ancestral genes of human and rhesus are identical, which means that no genes were lost within these regions over the past 25 Myr. Gene loss has occurred only in the youngest stratum (stratum 5), which comprises 3% of the human MSY and formed just before the divergence of the human and rhesus lineages [26]. These findings suggest that the human Y-linked genes have been stable and conserved, at least for the past 25 Myr.

Unique Sex Chromosomes and Mechanisms of Sex Determination - XO Males without SRY

Interestingly, complete loss of the Y chromosome has actually occurred in two rodent species of the genus *Tokudaia* and one species of the genus *Ellobius*. Globally, there are only three mammalian species, all of them placental mammals, with the surprising features of an XO/XO karyotype and no *SRY*. These apparently similar phenomena of loss of the Y chromosome and *SRY* were considered to have occurred independently during evolution because the genera *Ellobius* and *Tokudaia* are from different subfamilies, Arvicolonae and Murinae, respectively.

i) Ryukyu Spiny Rat, Genus Tokudaia

Ryukyu spiny rats belong to the genus *Tokudaia*, (Murinae, Muridae, Rodentia) and are mammals native to Japan. They are classified into three species, each of which is indigenous to only one island in southernmost Japan (Figure 3). *Tokudaia muenninki*, which lives on Okinawa-jima, has an XX/XY sex chromosome constitution, and a diploid chromosome number of $2n=44$ [27, 28]. However, the two other species, *Tokudaia osimensis* and *Tokudaia tokunoshimensis*, which live on Amami-Ohsima and Tokunoshima, respectively, have an XO/XO sex chromosome constitution owing to the absence of the Y chromosome. Consequently, *T. osimensis* and *T. tokunoshimensis* have odd numbers of diploid chromosomes: $2n=25$ and $2n=45$, respectively [29-31]. In addition, these XO species have no *SRY*. Although multiple *SRY* genes have been detected in males of *T. muenninki* (XY) by PCR and Southern blotting analysis, no *SRY* gene has been detected in these two XO species, *T. osimensis* and *T. tokunoshimensis* [28, 32, 33].

The *Tokudaia* genus is an interesting model for rapid and unique chromosome evolution. On the basis of molecular phylogenetic analysis, *T. muenninki* was shown to have been the first species in the genus to diverge [28], which suggests that the ancestral species of *Tokudaia* had a Y chromosome and *SRY*, and that loss of both the Y chromosome and *SRY* occurred in the common ancestor of *T. osimensis* and *T. tokunoshimensis* after they diverged from the common ancestor of all three *Tokudaia* species. In addition, after the divergence of *T. osimensis* and *T. tokunoshimensis*, centric fusion and tandem fusion occurred mainly in the lineage of *T. osimensis*, which resulted in a rapid decrease in chromosome number in this species.

The single X chromosomes of *T. osimensis* and *T. tokunoshimensis* are submetacentric and subtelocentric, respectively [29-31]. The gene orders of the X chromosomes were found to be conserved in the two species, whereas the position of the centromere on the X chromosome was found to differ by comparison of the gene order of the 22 X-linked genes [34]. This indicates that centromere repositioning occurred in the lineage of *T. osimensis*. Centromere repositioning is a recently discovered evolutionary phenomenon that involves the emergence of a new centromere along a chromosome and the inactivation of the old one, without chromosome rearrangement [35]. Centromere repositioning is not a very common evolutionary event; however, it has been suggested to have occurred in a number of eukaryotes.

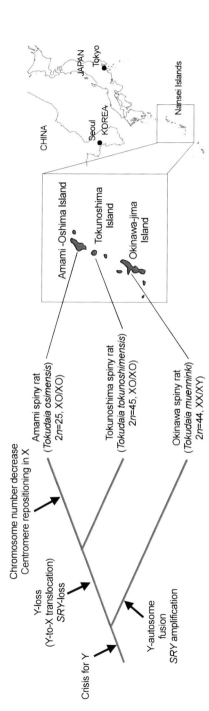

Figure 3. The evolution of *Tokudaia* together with the geographic distribution of *Tokudaia* species.

In addition, centromere repositioning provides a potentially powerful evolutionary force for reproductive isolation and speciation [36].

ii) Mole Vole, Genus Ellobius

The mole vole is a subterranean animal that belongs to the genus *Ellobius* (Arvicolinae, Cricetidae, Rodentia), which contains at least five species, namely, *Ellobius fuscocapillus* (geographical distribution: Baluchistan in Pakistan, Afghanistan, Iran, and Southern Turkmenistan), *Ellobius lutescens* (Armenia, Iran, Turkey, and Azerbaijian), the sister species *Ellobius tancrei* (Turkmenistan, Uzbekistan, Kazakhstan, and Xinjiang in Northwest China) and *Ellobius talpinus* (Ukraine, Crimea–Turkestan–Mongolia, Sinkiang, and Northern Afghanistan), and *Ellobius alaicus* [37]. Only *E. fuscocapillus* has an XX/XY karyotype, and the presence of *SRY* was demonstrated in the male genome of this species [38]. *Ellobius lutescens* has an odd number of chromosomes in both sexes: $2n=17$, XO/XO [39], with no *SRY* [38]; this species lives preferentially in semi-arid or grassland territories in riparian countries of the Caucasus Mountains [37, 40]. Interestingly, *E. tancrei*, *E. talpinus*, and *E. alaicus* have an XX/XX sex chromosome constitution [41, 42]; they vary in the number of autosomal chromosomes owing to Robertsonian fusion in *E. tancrei* and *E. talpinus* [43, 44]. The XO/XO and XX/XX species of *Ellobius* have no *SRY* [37], which suggests that the common ancestor of the *Ellobius* genus also possessed *SRY*, but that *SRY* was lost shortly after or during the divergence of the lineages of all extant *Ellobius* species.

Loss of the Y Chromosome Event in the XO Ryukyu Spiny Rat

It is known that the *SRY* gene was lost upon the disappearance of the Y chromosome in the XO Ryukyu spiny rat. What about other Y-linked genes? Studies revealed that the *RBMY1A1* gene, which is linked to the placental mammalian Y chromosome (see above section: The Y-linked genes – Sex determination and spermatogenesis), was also lost from the genome of the XO spiny rat [45]. *RBMY1A1* encodes a germ cell-specific nuclear protein [21, 22]. The similarity in amino acid sequences between RBMY1A1 and its X homologue, RBMX, is relatively low (48%). Thus, they have diverged functionally and *RBMY1A1* has been shown to be essential for spermatogenesis. Therefore, two important genes, *SRY* and *RBMY1A1*, which seem to be absolutely imperative for maleness, have been lost in the XO spiny rat. In addition, other proto-Y-linked genes were conserved in not only the male genome but also in the female genome as a result of their translocation from the Y chromosome to the distal end of the long arm of the X chromosome [45, 46]. Three stepwise events that led to the disappearance of the Y chromosome have been suggested: i) transposition of a few genes from the Y chromosome to autosomes, ii) the role of *SRY* being taken over by a new gene on an autosome, and iii) Y-to-X translocation of Y-linked genes. Of course, in most placental species, these Y-linked genes are expressed only in males, and two Y-linked genes, *EIF2S3Y* (eukaryotic translation initiation factor 2, subunit 3, structural gene Y-linked) and *KDM5D* (lysine (K)-specific demethylase 5D), have been shown to be expressed only in the male brain and testes of mice and humans. However, in the XO spiny rat, *T. osimensis*, these genes are expressed not only in male brain and testes but also in female brain and ovaries [45].

Avoidance of Loss of the Y Chromosome in the XY Spiny Rat

Tokudaia muenninki is the only species in the genus *Tokudaia* to retain the Y chromosome. As a consequence, it follows the general XY pattern of mammalian sex determination. However, the Y chromosome of *T. muenninki* has evolved in a unique manner. It is possible that the Y chromosome in the common ancestral species of the genus *Tokudaia* showed persistent instability. In the ancestral lineage common to the two XO/XO spiny rats, *T. osimensis* and *T. tokunoshimensis*, most of the Y-linked genes escaped to the X chromosome, and the Y chromosome was subsequently lost. In contrast, in the ancestral population of *T. muenninki*, the X and Y chromosomes fused with a pair of autosomes [47]. Such fusion is proposed because the X and Y chromosomes of *T. muenninki* are unusually large [27, 28]. The euchromatic regions of the X and Y chromosomes constitute 8% and 4% of the haploid genome, respectively (generally 5% and less than 2%, respectively), as the result of this autosomal fusion [28].

The enlargement of the Y chromosome through fusion with an autosome extended the pseudoautosomal regions (PARs) of the sex chromosomes. PARs behave like a pair of autosomes and recombine during male meiosis; this recombination is thought to play a critical role in spermatogenesis [48-50]. XY male mice with an inverted X PAR, or Y PAR flanked at the distal end by an X PAR boundary together with adjacent X-specific material, or both of the variant PARs are known to produce XO progeny by the production of unusual

X and Y products and consequent loss of the sex chromosome [51]. If a variant PAR was associated with the loss of the Y chromosome in an ancestral lineage common to the two XO/XO spiny rats, *T. osimensis* and *T. tokunoshimensis*, loss of the Y chromosome might have been avoided in the ancestral lineage of *T. muenninki* because the Y chromosome was stabilized by the acquisition of new PARs [47].

New Sex-Determining Gene That Substitutes for SRY

The mammalian sex-determining gene *SRY* is absent in the XO species of *Ellobius* and *Tokudaia*, which indicates that these species possess a novel sex-determining mechanism that is independent of this gene. In *E. lutescens*, genes with important functions in gonadal differentiation were analyzed by either segregation analysis of intragenic markers to show whether or not alleles segregate independently of sex or a sequence comparison between males and females. Dr. Walter Just and colleagues bred *E. lutescens* in captivity and some breeding pairs produced eleven offspring, with a litter size of up to six pups at intervals of four to six weeks [37]. Consequently, it was possible to use this cohort to investigate the inheritance of alleles in the offspring. The following X-linked genes were studied as putative sex-determining genes in *E. lutescens*: *ATRX* (alpha thalassemia/mental retardation syndrome X-linked), *NR0B1* (nuclear receptor subfamily 0, group B, member 1, also known as *DAX1*), and *SOX3*, and the autosome-linked genes: *AR* (androgen receptor), *DMRT1* (doublesex- and mab-3-related transcription factor 1), *FOXL2* (forkhead box L2), *NR5A1*, *PISRT1* (polled intersex syndrome-regulated transcript 1), and *SOX9*. All of these genes were ruled out as sex-determining factors because their alleles were shown to segregate independently of sex [37, 52-54]. The findings indicate that the single X chromosome of *E. lutescens* is not a sex chromosome any more, and a novel sex-determining factor might have developed on an autosome.

Comparative studies on the mechanisms of sex determination have revealed that the master control genes at the top of the regulatory hierarchy can change dramatically as new species and genera evolve, whereas the genes at the bottom of the hierarchy remain the same, carrying out essentially identical functions from one species to the next [55-57]. A model was proposed for the evolution of the sex-determining gene cascade by gene duplication, in which a second copy of a gene at the bottom of the hierarchy is produced by gene duplication and then the new copy acquires a novel function in sex determination [57]. The model fish species medaka (*Oryzias latipes*) provides evidence to support this hypothesis. Medaka is a small aquarium fish with the sex chromosome composition XX/XY. In this fish, a duplicate copy of the transcription factor dmrt1 (*dmY/dmrt1Y*: Y-linked doublesex- and mab-3-related transcription factor), which was derived from the autosomal linkage group 9, acquired a function as a master regulator of testicular development after it was inserted into the present Y chromosome [58, 59]. It is possible that a similar event occurred in the ancestor of the *Ellobius* and *Tokudaia* species that do not contain *SRY*; namely, a new copy of a gene, which emerged by duplication, might have acquired a new function as a sex-determining gene.

To identify candidate genes involved in male sex determination in *Tokudaia*, the copy numbers and chromosomal locations of 10 genes were examined in the two XO/XO species of *Tokudaia*, which lack an *SRY* gene [60]: *ATRX*, *CBX2* (chromobox 2; also known as *M33*), *DMRT1*, *FGF9* (fibroblast growth factor 9), *NR0B1*, *NR5A1*, *RSPO1* (R-spondin 1), *SOX9*, *WNT4* (wingless-related MMTV integration site 4), and *WT1* (Wilms tumor 1). These 10 genes are the most important genes for sexual development of the gonads. They have been implicated in human and mouse sexual development, and gain-of-function and/or loss-of-function mutations in these genes cause disorders of sexual development in mice and humans. The products of these genes function in the proximity (upstream and/or downstream) of the mammalian sex-determining gene, *SRY*. Southern blot analysis and fluorescence *in situ* hybridization mapping were performed to detect extra copies of these genes. *CBX2* was mapped to two loci in each of the two species (*T. osimensis*: 3q24, 6p11.2; *T. tokunoshimensis*: 10q25–q26, 14q12–q13.1). Furthermore, quantitative analysis of the gene in these two species by quantitative real-time PCR showed that *CBX2* was present in multiple copies in both sexes, and males had two or three more copies than females. *CBX2* is a member of the mammalian Polycom*b* group, which is required to repress *Hox* gene transcription at the chromatin level [61-63]. Mice in which *Cbx2* is knocked out are unique in showing hypoplastic gonad formation in both sexes and male-to-female sex reversal [64]. Among *Sry*-positive *Cbx2*-knockout mice, 50–70% are phenotypically normal females that have ovaries with follicles, a uterus, and normal external genitalia, which suggests that *Cbx2* deficiency might cause sex reversal [64]. A similar case has been reported in humans; namely, a girl with the karyotype 46,XY who had normal female external genitalia due to loss-of-function mutations in *CBX2* [65]. Collectively, these findings indicate that *Cbx2/CBX2* actively represses ovarian development [64, 65]. It is likely that these extra copies of *CBX2* in males repress ovarian development and hence cause the undifferentiated gonad to become testes in these species. Therefore, the differences in gene dosage might determine the developmental fate of the undifferentiated gonad in these species.

However, it might be difficult to confirm that *CBX2* is a new sex-determining gene because *Tokudaia* species are endangered and protected as natural treasures by Japanese law. As such, it is quite difficult to obtain an embryo at the developmental stage at which sex is determined. Successful breeding of *Tokudaia* animals in captivity has never been achieved. This means that there are insufficient samples to analyze the molecular mechanism of gonadal differentiation and the genetic inheritance of a candidate gene by offspring in a sex-dependent manner.

Conclusion

Studies that involve comparison between human and primate Y chromosomes suggest that the human Y-linked genes have been stable and conserved for at least the past 25 Myr. These empirical data on human Y-chromosome evolution seem to refute the hypothesis that the loss of human Y-linked genes is inexorable, and will lead to the disappearance of the human Y chromosome in the future. However, major and rapid chromosome rearrangement can sometimes occur within a short period of evolutionary time, if the right conditions prevail, for example, a population bottleneck, and so on. In fact, complete loss of the Y chromosome occurred independently in each lineage of the *Tokudaia* and *Ellobius*. Thus, it is likely that loss of the human Y chromosome will occur at some point in an individual, but it remains unclear whether this mutation would then spread and become fixed in the population. Furthermore, the cases of *Tokudaia* and *Ellobius* show us that loss of the Y chromosome need not lead to the extinction of a species, including humans. Instead, these cases show that mammals can lose the Y chromosome and still retain their maleness. Although the XO species of *Tokudaia* and *Ellobius* are exceptional animals, enlargement of the X and Y chromosomes owing to fusion with an autosome, as seen in *T. muenninki* (XX/XY), has also been reported in other mammalian species [66-70]. This rearrangement involves the acquisition of new sex chromosomes, and also results in expansion of the recombination region and an increase in the number of linked genes. In fact, most human Y-linked genes are relics of an autosomal addition [71]. The PAR of placental mammals arose as part of a larger autosomal addition to the X and Y chromosomes that occurred 130–80 MYR ago [72] (Figure 1). Enlargement of the Y chromosome by the addition of an autosome could be an important chromosomal rearrangement to stabilize X-Y pairing, and one mechanism by which the Y chromosome could be retained.

References

[1] Ohno, S. (1967). *Sex Chromosomes and Sex-linked Genes*. Berlin: Springer Verlag.

[2] Charlesworth, B. (1991) The evolution of sex chromosomes. *Science*, 251, 1030-1033.

[3] Lahn, B. T. and Page, D. C. (1999) Four evolutionary strata on the human X chromosome. *Science*, 286, 964-967.

[4] Ross, M. T., Grafham, D. V., Coffey, A. J., et al. (2005) The DNA sequence of the human X chromosome. *Nature*, 434, 325-337.

[5] Charlesworth, B. and Charlesworth, D. (2000) The degeneration of Y chromosomes. *Philos. Trans. R. Soc. Lond. B Biol. Sci.*, 355, 1563-1572.

[6] Hughes, J. F. and Rozen, S. (2012) Genomics and genetics of human and primate Y chromosomes. *Annu. Rev. genomics Hum. Genet.*, 13, 3.1-3.26.

[7] Graves, J. A. M. (2006) Sex chromosome specialization and degeneration in mammals. *Cell*, 124, 901-914.

[8] Aitken, R. J. and Graves, J. A. M. (2002) The future of sex. *Nature*, 415, 963.

[9] Ferguson-Smith, M. A. (1966) X-Y chromosomal interchange in the aetiology of true hermaphroditism and of XX Klinefelter's syndrome. *Lancet*, 2, 475-476.

[10] Ferguson-Smith, M. A. and Affara, N. A. (1988) Accidental X-Y recombination and the aetiology of XX males and true hermaphrodites. *Philos. Trans. R. Soc. Lond. B Biol. Sci.*, 322, 133-144.

[11] Sinclair, A. H., Berta, P., Palmer, M. S., Hawkins, J. R., Griffiths, B. L., Smith, M. J., Foster, J. W., Frischauf, A. M., Lovell-Badge, R., Goodfellow, P. N. (1990) A gene from the human sex-determining region encodes a protein with homology to a conserved DNA-binding motif. *Nature*, 346, 240-244.

[12] Berta, P., Hawkins, J. R., Sinclair, A. H., Taylor, A., Griffiths, B. L., Goodfellow, P. N., Fellous, M. (1990) Genetic evidence equating SRY and the testis-determining factor. *Nature*, 348, 448-450.

[13] Jäger, R. J., Anvret, M., Hall, K., Scherer, G. (1990) A human XY female with a frame shift mutation in the candidate testis-determining gene SRY. *Nature,* 348, 452-454.
[14] Gubbay, J., Collignon, J., Koopman, P., Capel, B., Economou, A., Münsterberg, A., Vivian, N., Goodfellow, P., Lovell-Badge, R. (1990) A gene mapping to the sex-determining region of the mouse Y chromosome is a member of a novel family of embryonically expressed genes. *Nature,* 346, 245-250.
[15] Koopman, P., Gubbay, J., Vivian, N., Goodfellow, P., Lovell-Badge, R. (1991) Male development of chromosomally female mice transgenic for Sry. *Nature,* 351, 117-121.
[16] Sekido, R. and Lovell-Badge, R. (2008) Sex determination involves synergistic action of SRY and SF1 on a specific Sox9 enhancer. *Nature,* 453, 930-934.
[17] Wilhelm, D., Palmer, S., Koopman, P. (2007) Sex determination and gonadal development in mammals. *Physiol Rev.,* 87, 1-28.
[18] Waters, P.D., Wallis, M.C., Marshall Graves, J. A. (2007) Mammalian sex--Origin and evolution of the Y chromosome and SRY. *Semin. Cell Dev. Biol.,* 18, 389-400.
[19] Lahn, B. T. and Page, D. C. (1999). Four evolutionary strata on the human X chromosome. *Nature,* 286, 964-967.
[20] Salido, E. C., Yen, P. H., Koprivnikar, K., Yu, L. C., Shapiro, L. J. (1992) The human enamel protein gene amelogenin is expressed from both the X and the Y chromosomes. *Am. J. Hum. Genet.,* 50, 303-316.
[21] Mazeyrat, S., Saut, N., Mattei, M. G., Mitchell, M. J. (1999) RBMY evolved on the Y chromosome from a ubiquitously transcribed X-Y identical gene. *Nat. Genet.,* 22, 224-226.
[22] Elliott, D. J. (2004) The role of potential splicing factors including RBMY, RBMX, hnRNPG-T and STAR proteins in spermatogenesis. *Int. J. Androl.,* 27, 328-334.
[23] Hughes, J. F., Skaletsky, H., Pyntikova, T., Minx, P. J., Graves, T., Rozen, S., Wilson, R. K., Page, D. C. (2005) Conservation of Y-linked genes during human evolution revealed by comparative sequencing in chimpanzee. *Nature,* 437, 100-103.
[24] Kuroki, Y., Toyoda, A., Noguchi, H., Taylor, T. D., Itoh, T., Kim, D. S., Kim, D. W., Choi, S. H., Kim, I. C., Choi, H. H., Kim, Y. S., Satta, Y., Saitou, N., Yamada, T., Morishita, S., Hattori, M., Sakaki, Y., Park, H. S., Fujiyama, A. (2006) Comparative analysis of chimpanzee and human

Y chromosomes unveils complex evolutionary pathway. *Nat. Genet.*, 38, 158-167.
[25] Hughes, J. F., Skaletsky, H., Pyntikova, T., Graves, T. A., van Daalen, S. K., Minx, P. J., Fulton, R. S., McGrath, S. D., Locke, D. P., Friedman, C., Trask, B. J., Mardis, E. R., Warren, W. C., Repping, S., Rozen, S., Wilson, R. K., Page, D. C. (2010) Chimpanzee and human Y chromosomes are remarkably divergent in structure and gene content. *Nature*, 463, 536-539.
[26] Hughes, J. F., Skaletsky, H., Brown, L. G., Pyntikova, T., Graves, T., Fulton, R. S., Dugan, S., Ding, Y., Buhay, C. J., Kremitzki, C., Wang, Q., Shen, H., Holder, M., Villasana, D., Nazareth, L. V., Cree, A., Courtney, L., Veizer, J., Kotkiewicz, H., Cho, T. J., Koutseva, N., Rozen, S., Muzny, D. M., Warren, W. C., Gibbs, R. A., Wilson, R. K., Page, D. C. (2012) Strict evolutionary conservation followed rapid gene loss on human and rhesus Y chromosomes. *Nature*, 483, 82-86.
[27] Tsuchiya, K., Wakana, S., Suzuki, H., Hattori, S., Hayashi, Y. (1989) Taxonomic study of Tokudaia (Rodentia: Muridae): I. Genetic differentiation. *Memoirs. Nat. Sci. Museum*, Tokyo, 22, 227-234.
[28] Murata, C., Yamada, F., Kawauchi, N., Matsuda, Y., Kuroiwa, A. (2010) Multiple copies of SRY on the large Y chromosome of the Okinawa spiny rat, Tokudaia muenninki. *Chromosome Res.*, 18, 623-634.
[29] Honda, T., Suzuki, H., Itoh, M. (1977) An unusual sex chromosome constitution found in the Amami spinous country-rat, Tokudaia osimensis osimensis. *Jpn. J. Genet.*, 52, 247-249.
[30] Honda, T., Suzuki, H., Itoh, M., Hayashi, K. (1978) Karyotypical differences of the Amami spinous country-rats, Tokudaia osimensis osimensis obtained from two neighbouring islands. *Jpn. J. Genet.*, 53, 297-299.
[31] Kobayashi, T., Yamada, F., Hashimoto, T., Abe, S., Matsuda, Y. Kuroiwa, A. (2007) Exceptional minute sex-specific region in the X0 mammal, Ryukyu spiny rat. *Chromosome Res.*, 15, 175-187.
[32] Soullier, S., Hanni, C., Catzeflis, F., Berta, P., Laudet, V. (1998) Male sex determination in the spiny rat Tokudaia osimensis (Rodentia: Muridae) is not Sry dependent. *Mamm. Genome*, 9, 590-592.
[33] Sutou, S., Mitsui, Y., Tsuchiya, K. (2001) Sex determination without the Y chromosome in two Japanese rodents Tokudaia osimensis osimensis and Tokudaia osimensis spp. *Mamm. Genome*, 12, 17-21.

[34] Kobayashi, T., Yamada, F., Hashimoto, T., Abe, S., Matsuda, Y. (2008) Centromere repositioning in the X chromsome of XO/XO mammals, Ryukyu spiny rat. *Chromoosme Res.*, 16:587-593.

[35] Montefalcone, G., Tempesta, S., Rocchi, M., Archidiacono, N. (1999) Centromere repositioning. *Genome Res.*, 12, 1184-1188.

[36] Rocchi, M., Archidiacono, N., Schempp, W., Capozzi, O., Stanyon, R. (2012) Centromere repositioning in mammals. (2012) *Heredity*, 108, 59-67.

[37] Just, W., Baumstark, A., Süss, A., Graphodatsky, A., Rens, W., Schäfer, N., Bakloushinskaya, I., Hameister, H., Vogel, W. (2007) Ellobius lutescens: sex determination and sex chromosome. *Sex Dev.*, 1, 211-221.

[38] Just, W., Rau, W., Vogel, W., Akhverdian, M., Fredga, K., Graves, J. A., Lyapunova, E. (1995) *Absence of Sry in species of the vole Ellobius.* 11, 117-118.

[39] Matthey, R. (1953) La formule chromosomique et le problém de la détermination sexuelle chez Ellobius lutescens Thomas (Rodentia-Muridae-Microtinae). *Arch Klaus-Shift Verteb-Forsch*, 28, 65-73.

[40] Coskun, Y. (2001) On distribution, morphology and biology of the mole vole, Ellobius lutescens Thomas, 1897 (Mammalia: Rodentia) in eastern *Turkey. Zool. Middle East*, 23, 5-12.

[41] Kolomiets, O. L., Vorontsov, N. N., Lyapunova, E. A., Mazurova, T. F. (1991) Ultrastructure, meiotic behavior, and evolution of sex chromosomes of the genus Ellobius. *Genetica*, 84, 179-189.

[42] Romanenko, S. A. and Volobouev, V. (2012) Non-Sciuromorph Rodent Karyotypes in Evolution. *Cytogenet. Genome Res.* [Epub ahead of print]

[43] Ginatulin, A. A., Ginautulina, L. K., Borrissov, Y. M., Lyapunova, E. A., Vorontsov, N. N. (1977) Relationship between the study of DNA reassociation kinetics of various chromosomal forms of Ellobius and questions concerning the pathways of chromosome rearrangement during evolution. *Mol. Biol.* (Mosk), 11, 883-890.

[44] Borissov, T. M., Lyapunova, E. A., Vorontsov, N. N. (1991) Karyotype evolution in the genus Ellobius (Microtinae, Rodentia). *Genetica,* 27, 523-532.

[45] Kuroiwa, A., Ishiguchi, Y., Yamada, F., Abe, S., Matsuda, Y. (2010) The process of a Y-loss event in an XO/XO mammal, the Ryukyu spiny rat. *Chromosoma*, 119, 519-526.

[46] Arakawa, Y., Nishida-Umehara, C., Matsuda, Y., Sutou, S., Suzuki, H. (2002) X-chromosomal localization of mammalian Y-linked genes in

two XO species of the Ryukyu spiny rat. *Cytogenet. Genome Res.*, 99, 303-309.
[47] Murata, C., Yamada, F., Kawauchi, N., Matsuda, Y., Kuroiwa, A. (2012) The Y chromosome of the Okinawa spiny rat, Tokudaia muenninki, was rescued through fusion with an autosome. *Chromosome Res.*, 20, 111-125.
[48] Kauppi, L., Barchi, M., Baudat, F., Romanienko, P. J., Keeney, S., Jasin, M. (2011) Distinct properties of the XY pseudoautosomal region crucial for male meiosis. *Science,* 331, 916-920.
[49] Matsuda, Y., Moens, P. B., Chapman, V. M. (1992) Deficiency of X and Y chromosomal pairing at meiotic prophase in spermatocytes of sterile interspecific hybrids between laboratory mice (Mus domesticus) and Mus spretus. *Chromosoma,* 101, 483-492.
[50] Mohandas, T. K., Speed, R. M., Passage, M. B., Yen, P. H., Chandley, A. C., Shapiro, L. J. (1992) Role of the pseudoautosomal region in sex-chromosome pairing during male meiosis: meiotic studies in a man with a deletion of distal Xp. *Am. J. Hum. Genet.,* 51, 526-533.
[51] Burgoyne, P. S. and Evans, E. P. (2000) A high frequency of XO offspring from X(Paf)Y* male mice: evidence that the Paf mutation involves an inversion spanning the X PAR boundary. *Cytogenet. Cell Genet.,* 91, 57-61.
[52] Mashal, R. D., Koontz, J., Sklar, J. (1995) Detection of mutation by cleavage of DNA heteroduplexes with bacteriophage resolves. *Nat. Genet.,* 9, 177-183.
[53] Baumstark, A., Akhverdyan, M., Schulze, A., Reisert, I., Vogel, W., Just, W. (2001) Exclusion of SOX9 as the testis determining factor in Ellobius lutescens: evidence for another testis determining gene besides SRY and SOX9. *Mol. Genet. Metab.*, 72, 61-66.
[54] Baumstark, A., Hameister, H., Hakhverdyan, M., Bakloushinskaya, I., Just, W. (2005) Characterization of Pisrt1/Fox12 in Ellobius lutescens and exclusion as sex-determining genes. *Mamm. Genome.*, 16, 281-289.
[55] Graham, P., Penn, J. K. M., Schedl, P. (2002) Masters change, slaves remain. *Bioessays,* 25, 1-4
[56] Wilkins, A. S. (1995) Moving up the hierarchy: a hypothesis on the evolution of a genetic sex determination pathway. *Bioessays,* 17, 71-77.
[57] Schartl, M. (2004) Sex chromosome evolution in non-mammalian vertebrates. *Curr. Opin. Genet. Dev.*, 14, 634-641.
[58] Matsuda, M., Nagahama, Y., Shinomiya, A., Sato, T., Matsuda, C., Kobayashi, T., Morrey, C. E., Shibata, N., Asakawa, S., Shimizu, N.,

Hori, H., Hamaguchi, S., Sakaizumi, M. (2002) DMY is a Y-specific DM-domain gene required for male development in the medaka fish. *Nature,* 417, 559-563.
[59] Nanda, I., Kondo, M., Hornung, U., Asakawa, S., Winkler, C., Shimizu, A., Shan, Z., Haaf, T., Shimizu, N., Shima, A., Schmid, M., Schartl, M. (2002) A duplicated copy of DMRT1 in the sex-determining region of the Y chromosome of the medaka, Oryzias latipes. *Proc. Natl. Acad. Sci. USA.,* 99, 11778-11783.
[60] Kuroiwa, A., Handa, S., Nishiyama, C., Chiba, E., Yamada, F., Abe, S., Matsuda, Y. (2011) Additional copies of CBX2 in the genomes of males of mammals lacking SRY, the Amami spiny rat (Tokudaia osimensis) and the Tokunoshima spiny rat (Tokudaia tokunoshimensis). *Chromosome Res,* 19, 635-644.
[61] Pearce, J. J., Singh, P. B., Graunt, S. J. (1992) The mouse has a Polycomb-like chromobox gene. *Development,* 114, 921-929.
[62] Paro, R., Hogness, D. S. (1991) The Polycomb protein shares a homologous domain with a heterochromatin-associated protein of Drosophila. *Proc. Natl. Acad. Sci. USA.,* 88, 263-267.
[63] Pirrotta, V. (1997) Chromatin-silencing mechanisms in Drosophila maintain patterns of gene expression. *Trends. Genet.,* 13, 314-318.
[64] Katoh-Fukui, Y., Tsuchiya, R., Shiroishi, T., Nakahara, Y., Hashimoto, N., Noguchi, K., Higashinakagawa, T. (1998) Male-to-female sex reversal in M33 mutant mice. *Nature,* 393, 688-692.
[65] Biason-Lauber, A., Konrad, D., Meyer, M., DeBeaufort, C., Schoenle, E. J. (2009) Ovaries and female phenotype in a girl with 46,XY karyotype and mutations in the CBX2 gene. *Am. J. Hum. Genet,* 84, 658-663.
[66] Deuve, J. L., Bennett, N. C., O'Brien, P. C. M., Ferguson-Smith, M. A., Faulkes, C. G., Britton-Davidian, J., Robinson, T. J. (2006) Complex evolution of X and Y autosomal translocations in the giant mole-rat, Cryptomys mechowi (Bathyergidae). *Chromosome Res.,* 14, 681-691.
[67] Veyrunes, F., Catalan, J., Sicard, B. Robinson, T. J., Duplantier, J. M., Granjon, L., Dobigny, G., Britton-Davidian, J. (2004) Autosome and sex chromosome diversity among the African pygmy mice, subgenus Nannomys (Murinae; Mus). *Chromosome Res.,* 12, 369–382.
[68] Veyrunes, F., Catalan, J., Tatard, C., Cellier-Holzem, E., Watson, J., Chevret, P., Robinson, T. J., Britton-Davidian, J. (2010) Mitochondrial and chromosomal insights into karyotypic evolution of the pygmy mouse, Mus minutoides, in South Africa. *Chromosome Res.,* 18, 563-574.

[69] Gallagher, D. S., Davis, S. K., De Donato, M., Burzlaff, J. D., Womack, J. E., Taylor, J. F., Kumamoto, A. T. (1998) A karyotypic analysis of nilgai, Boselaphus tragocamelus (Artiodactyla: Bovidae). *Chromosome Res.*, 6, 505-513.

[70] Rubes, J., Kubickova, S., Pagacova, E., Cernohorska, H., Di Berardino, D., Antoninova, M., Vahala, J., Robinson, T. J. (2008) Phylogenomic study of spiral-horned antelope by cross-species chromosome painting. *Chromosome Res.*, 16, 935-947.

[71] Waters, P. D., Duffy, B., Frost, C. J., Delbridge, M. L., Graves, J. A. (2001) The human Y chromosome derives largely from a single autosomal region added to the sex chromosomes 80-130 million years ago. Cytogenet. *Cell Genet.,* 92, 74-79.

[72] Toder, R. and Graves, J. A. (1998) CSF2RA, ANT3, and STS are autosomal in marsupials: implications for the origin of the pseudoautosomal region of mammalian sex chromosomes. *Mamm. Genome*, 9, 373-376.

In: Sex Chromosomes: New Research ISBN: 978-1-62417-143-7
Editors: M. D'Aquino and V. Stallone © 2013 Nova Science Publishers, Inc.

Chapter IV

The Role of Y Chromosome Genes on Tumor Development Risk in Disgenetic Gonads

Monica Vannucci Nunes Lipay[1,2] and Bianca Bianco[3]
[1]Associate Professor, Jundiaí Medical College, SP, Brazil
[2]UNIFESP, SP, Brazil
[3]Division of Human Reproduction and Genetics,
Department of Gynecology and Obstetrics,
Faculdade de Medicina do ABC, Santo André/SP-Brazil

Abstract

The presence of Y-chromosome material in patients with dysgenetic gonads increases the risk of gonadal tumors, especially gonadoblastoma (GB). In 1987, Page hypothesized that there is a locus, termed GBY (gonadoblastoma on the Y chromosome), which predisposes the dysgenetic gonads to developing such *in situ* tumors. Studies have been suggested that the testis-specific protein Y encoded (TSPY) repeated gene is the putative region for this oncogenic locus, and could potentially be involved in other human cancers. Hildenbrand et al. studied a patient with TS and a 45,X/46,X,mar karyotype who developed unilateral gonadoblastoma. Cytogenetic and molecular studies confirmed that the marker was derived from a Y chromosome. The authors investigated the gonadal material by immunohistochemistry for the expression of the

TSPY gene, and the results revealed a high level of TSPY protein expression. However, one of the Y sequences most frequently used in Turner Syndrome (TS) patients screening is the *SRY* gene, because of its localization and its important role in the signaling cascade of sex determining events.

It is already well established that the presence of Y-chromosome material in patients with dysgenetic gonads increases the risk of gonadal tumors, such as gonadoblastoma and dysgerminoma, or of nontumoral androgen-producing lesions. This confers clinical importance to the detection of the Y-chromosome mosaicism in TS.

Screening for Y-chromosome specific sequences is important in the follow-up of TS patients, considering that it is correlated to the proven risk of gonadal tumors development. Thus, the early detection of such events could be of great importance to preventing of gonadal tumor development in TS patients.

The *SRY* gene plays a pivotal role in the signaling chain that occurs during embryonic development, functioning as an activator and also being regulated by several genes. Moreover, it is of fundamental importance in cell differentiation and, consequently, in the determination of the gonadal microenvironment, which starts interacting in the presence of androgens. This way, genes that perform in sex differentiation and development would have an altered expression in the dysgenetic gonads of TS patients, possibily implying in gonadal tumorigenesis. Significant difference in the dysgenetic and controls gonads regarding the expression of genes *OCT4*, *SRY*, and *TSPY* in both gonads of a case characterized by temporal exposure of dysgenetic gonads to the Y-chromosome sequences. This fact could lead to neoplastic development as a result of accumulated modifications in the gonadal microenvironment, especially under the hormonal activity that characterizes the pubertal period, even in the absence of histopathologic abnormalities of the gonads.

Y Chromosome: An Overview

Y chromosomes have evolved independently in multiple groups of animals and plants and consequently are bewilderingly diverse. However, all Y chromosomes share two defining features: restriction to the male germ line and limited recombination with a homologous partner during meiosis. Only the Y chromosomes of human and two of our closest relatives—chimpanzee and rhesus macaque—have been completely sequenced at the present time. [1]

It has been known for half a century that in mammals a Y chromosome is required for male sex determination. Genomic studies of the human Y chromosome since the 1980s, which culminated in the publication of the complete human Y-chromosome sequence in 2003. However, because the highly repetitive nature of Y chromosomes makes them tremendously difficult to sequence, they have lagged behind in the genomics revolution.

The human Y chromosome is heterogeneous, consisting of five highly distinct types of sequences: pseudoautosomal, heterochromatic, X-transposed, X-degenerate, and ampliconic.

The pseudoautosomal regions are located at the extreme termini of the Y and X chromosomes and constitute a small fraction of the total Y-chromosome sequence.[1] During meiosis, recombination between the Y and X chromosomes is normally restricted to these regions. Notably, the human Y chromosome is the only Y chromosome characterized thus far with a second pseudoautosomal region. The remainder of the Y chromosome, the MSY (Male Specific region of Y chromosome), has no partner for homologous recombination and is transmitted clonally, from father to son, solely through the male germ line.

A significant fraction of the human MSY comprises several discrete blocks of heterochromatic sequence, including a single ~40-Mb mass of heterochromatin on the long arm. More recently, however, several genes and mutations in the MSY have been definitively tied to human disease. These successes relied mainly on molecular-genetic and genomic approaches, and in the study of MSY mutations that affect spermatogenesis, they depended critically on the availability of the complete and accurate sequence of the human MSY's ampliconic regions. [1]

There are additional functional findings about the human MSY that are either preliminary or of specialized interest. First, one report found an association between the gr/gr deletion and testicular germ-cell tumors. [1]

Second, the presence of all or part of the Y chromosome in women (for example, in XY females with gonadal dysgenesis or women with Turner syndrome who are mosaic for 45, X and 46,XY cells) predisposes to a relatively benign germ-cell tumor, gonadoblastoma. [1, 2]

Third, multiple X-degenerate genes encode H-Y antigens. [1] These antigens are involved in (*a*) rejection of male grafts by female recipients and (*b*) immune response by engrafted female donor cells against a male host. The latter can cause both graft-versus-host disease and graft-versus-leukemia activity. [1]

The Sex-determining Factor: Searching for the *SRY* Gene

Not until 1959 did researchers realize that the human Y chromosome must bear a dominant, testis-determining gene—a gene that, when present, causes the embryonic gonad to develop into a testis. Thirty years later, this gene and its mouse ortholog were identified and dubbed *SRY* (for *sex determining region Y*).

The approximate location of *SRY* was initially inferred based on analysis of naturally occurring genomic translocations and deletions. [3] These included translocations of the tip of the Y chromosome (which contains *SRY*) to the X chromosome, resulting in XX males. Complementary evidence for the location of *SRY* came from the feminizing effects of deletions of the distal short arm of the Y chromosome. Eventually these investigations led to the cloning of *SRY* in human and mouse. [1]

Male sex determination in most mammals is initiated by the *SRY* (sex-determining region on the Y chromosome) gene, expression of which in pre-Sertoli cells drives the differentiation of the bipotential embryonic genital ridges towards testis commitment. *SRY* protein binds to the TESCO (testis-specific enhancer of Sox9 core) element of Sox9 and activates the expression of this crucial downstream target.

In turn, SOX9 protein orchestrates the genetic cascade of testis development. In line with a function of SRY proteins as sequence-specific transcription factors, all SRY proteins identified to date include an evolutionarily conserved HMG (high-mobility group) DNA-binding domain, which has taken center stage in research into *SRY* structure, function and evolution.

The HMG box is the signature domain of the *SOX* (*SRY*-type HMG box) family of transcription factors. It has attracted much of the research attention since Sry was identified as the male sex-determining gene, perhaps because it is highly conserved among SRY proteins from different species. This 79 amino-acid domain contains two nuclear localization signals that allow SRY to access the cell nucleus, and provides the structural basis of SRY's ability to bind and bend DNA. Nevertheless, all SRY proteins contain additional regions outside the HMG box, albeit sharing much less sequence homology between different species. [4]

The Progression of Sexual Differentiation

In mammals, sexually dimorphic establishment of the reproductive system follows three distinct steps. Initial sex determination (also known as chromosomal sex determination) occurs at the time of fertilization when sperm carrying either a Y or X chromosome fuses with the X chromosome-bearing oocyte. Once sex chromosome composition of the embryos is established (XY vs. XX), the second step (primary or gonadal sex determination) proceeds, in which the gonadal structure (testis or ovary) is specified. The sex-determining gene on the Y chromosome (*SRY*) is both necessary and sufficient to initiate testis morphogenesis. On the other hand, in the XX embryo, the absence of the *SRY* gene results in the initial formation of the ovary. Following the establishment of the gonad, the final stage of sex differentiation (or secondary sex determination) occurs when sex-specific development of the reproductive tracts and external genitalia are completed.

Initially, the Wolffian and Müllerian ducts, the precursors of the male and female reproductive tracts, respectively, develop in both male and female embryos. In male embryos, the testes produce anti-Müllerian hormone (AMH) and testosterone, which cause Müllerian duct regression and differentiation of the Wolffian duct into the epididymis, vas deferens, and seminal vesicles, respectively. Female embryos do not produce these hormones, and therefore, the Wolffian duct regresses and the Müllerian duct is maintained and forms the oviduct, uterus, cervix, and upper part of the vagina. Androgens produced by the testes also masculinize the male external genitalia, and the absence of androgens in female leads to the development of female genitalia. This three-step sexual differentiation process is clearly initiated by sex chromosomes and its components. However, downstream morphogenetic events, such as the appearance of gonad-specific cell types and structure, reproductive tract differentiation, and external genitalia establishment, require intricate interactions between systemic endocrine and local signaling pathways. [5]

Disorders of Sex Development (DSD)

The group of developmental anomalies, referred to as DSD, previously referred to as intersex, is defined as conditions of incomplete or disordered genital or gonadal development leading to a discordance between genetic sex (i.e.,determined by the chromosomal constitution, of the X and Y chromosomes), gonadal sex (the testicular or ovarian development of the gonad) and phenotypic sex (the physical appearance of the individual). Recently, a revised classification system has been proposed, with the aim to reduce uncertainties on description. [6] The classification system is primarily based on the karyotype of the patient, resulting in three entities: (1) sex chromosomal DSD, (2) 46,XY DSD and (3) 46,XX DSD. The first group includes all patients with numerical sex chromosomal anomalies, such as 47,XXY (Klinefelter syndrome and variants), 45,X (Turner syndrome and variants), 45,X/46,XY (mixed gonadal dysgenesis) and 46,XX/46,XY (chimaerism). [6]

The 46, XY DSD group include all patients with (A) disorders of gonadal (testicular) development, including (1) complete and partial gonadal dysgenesis (due to mutation of *SRY, SOX9, SF1, WT1*, etc), (2) ovotesticular DSD and (3) testis regression; (B) disorders in androgen synthesis or action, including (1) disorders of androgen synthesis, (2) action and (C) others. [6, 7]

The 46, XX DSD group includes all patients with (A) disorders of gonadal (ovarian) development, including (1) gonadal dysgenesis, (2) ovotesticular DSD and (3) testicular DSD (i.e., *SRY* presence, duplication *SOX9* and mutation *RSPO1*); (B) androgen excess, including (1) foetal, (2) foetaplacental, (3) maternal and (C) others. Patients with the same phenotypical characteristics can be part of a different category due to the karyotype used for the primary sub-classification. In addition, patients might also switch from category, for example, based on additional information gathered, such as presence of mosaicisms. This might be a limitation in some cases. However, the consensus report must be interpreted as a living document, which at least allows a better description of the various types of disorders than the previous nomenclatures. It, therefore, allows a more straight forward sub-classification and correlative analyses, including investigation of the risk for malignant transformation of germ cells. [6]

Turner Syndrome (TS): A Constant Challenge for Clinical Management

Turner's syndrome (TS) is one of the most common cytogenetic abnormalities (1:2,500 among newborn females); it is compatible with life, even though the great majority of the conceptuses with the syndrome are spontaneously aborted. The syndrome is characterized by gonadal dysgenesis with primary amenorrhea, sexual infantilism, webbing of the neck, cubitus valgus, and short stature in phenotypic women. [8]

The etiology of this syndrome has been associated with total or partial monosomy of the X chromosome. Typically, besides the 45,X cell line, another cell line with a complete chromosome number, yet with one structurally abnormal X or Y chromosome, is observed. [2, 8]

The percentage of mosaicism with a cell line containing a normal or abnormal Y chromosome in TS has been estimated by cytogenetic analysis as being 5.5%. Conventional cytogenetic analysis may not detect structurally abnormal chromosomes if they are small or rare. In addition, approximately half of the unidentifiable marker chromosomes that occur with an estimated frequency of 3% in TS are Y-chromosome derived. [8, 9] Moreover, mosaicism may not be detected in peripheral blood but may be significant in samples from other tissues. Possible reasons for failure to detect Y-chromosome mosaicism by routine cytogenetic analysis include low-frequency mosaicism, small nonfluorescent marker chromosomes, translocation of Y material onto the X chromosome or autosomes, instability of chromosomes with structural aberrations, and mosaicism that is restricted to certain tissues. [8, 9, 10]

It is well established that the presence of Y-chromosome material in patients with dysgenetic gonads increases the risk of gonadal tumors, such as gonadoblastoma and dysgerminoma, or of nontumoral androgen-producing lesions. [7, 8, 9, 10, 11] This makes the detection of Y-chromosome mosaicism in TS of crucial clinical importance. [9, 11]

Gonadal Dysgenesis and Tumor Risk

Various types of human germ cell tumors (GCTs) can be found referred to as type I, II and III. The type I are the teratomas and yolk sac tumors of neonates and infants. Type II GCTs are the seminomas and nonseminomas, derived from carcinoma *in situ* (CIS)/intratubular germ cell neoplasia unclassified (ITGCNU). CIS/ITGCNU and seminoma cells mimic primordial germ cells/gonocytes, amongst others characterized by expression of the diagnostic marker OCT3/4-POU5F1. All invasive tumors show gain of the short arm of chromosome 12. The types III GCTs, i.e. spermatocytic seminomas, occur predominantly in elderly and only in the testis and originate from primary spermatocytes. Besides familial predisposition and infertility, disorders of sex differentiation (DSD) are a risk factor for type II GCTs. The type II GCTs are in fact an embryonic cancer in adult patients. This explains a number of specific characteristics, like their histology (totipotency), overall sensitivity to DNA-damaging agents, as well as their chromosomal and genetic constitution. [6]

Abnormalities in gonad organogenesis can lead to the development of gonadal tumors, especially in patients with dysgenetic gonads. Patients with disorders of sexual development are at increased risk of developing tumors originating from germ lines, also known as germ-cell tumors. Several risk factors have been identified for these kinds of germ-cell tumors, particularly those relating to gonads, including cryptorchidism and gonadal dysgenesis. [2, 7]

The precursor lesion for dysgenetic gonad tumors is named gonadoblastoma. This has the potential to progress towards invasive germ cell tumors, particularly dysgerminoma, and, less frequently, towards components of other tumors, such as embryonic carcinoma, teratoma, yolk sac tumor and choriocarcinoma. [7]

Gonadoblastoma is a mixed tumor of undifferentiated cells that recapitulates gonadal development and is able to originate dysgerminoma in 60% of the cases. Hyperandrogenism is a phenomenon commonly associated with gonadoblastoma, especially in cases of coexistence with dysgerminoma. [2]

There is strong evidence that gonadoblastoma results from a disorder in germ cell maturation. This model is supported by epidemiological and morphological observations, such as the presence of immunohistochemical germ cell markers (placental alkaline phosphatase) and proto-oncogenes (*KIT*). [2]

The genes *SRY* and *DYZ3* are the sequences most commonly used in studies. Controversy still exists regarding which Y-chromosome markers are the most relevant. In general, the *SRY* gene is the sequence most used, because of its location and important role in the sex differentiation cascade. [11]

However, with the identification of novel genes on the Y chromosome and the so-far unconfirmed suspicion that there is a specific gene associated with the development of gonadoblastoma, other regions have been associated with the development of this tumor.

Studies of Rutgers and Scully and Verp and Simpson [2] show that, among patients with gonadal dysgenesis and Y chromosome, gonadal tumor gonadoblastoma is the most frequent, ranging from 9 to 30% of cases. This neoplasm is composed of germ cells intimately mixed with cords of sex cells in groups or nests bounded, usually with a hyaline basement membrane, and focal or diffuse calcifications. [2]

Approximately 80% of patients with gonadoblastoma are phenotypically female. [3] Although gonadoblastomas were not metastatic tumors, other types of germ cell tumors could be associated with them. In fact, approximately 50% of tumor cells invaded the stroma and form a dysgerminoma, a term synonymous with the seminoma. About 17% of germinomas arising from gonadoblastomas are bilateral. [7]

In a study of 15 patients with gonadal dysgenesis and female phenotype, Wallace and Levin [2] observed the occurrence of gonadal tumors in seven of them. Among the gonads that showed malignancies, there were five gonadoblastomas, four disgerminomas and a malignant neoplasm of intratubular germ cell. One of the patients also showed a gonadal stromal tumor.

Gonadoblastomas are found almost exclusively (96%) in dysgenetic gonads of 46, XY individuals, but also have been observed rarely in individuals without the Y chromosome (three cases with karyotype 46, XX, a 45, X, two 45, X / 46, XX, four with structural abnormalities of X, a 46, XX, del (11p) and two true hermaphrodites. [4]

In a series of 13 patients with gonadoblastoma, found from the pathological diagnosis, five were male and of these, 3 (46, XY) were brothers who had bilateral cryptorchidism and also presented Müllerian derivatives, a [46, X, + mar (Y+)] and one had bilateral cryptorchidism (karyotype unknown) had seminoma and focal calcification, and uterus and fallopian tubes. Of the eight female patients, one was a carrier of pure gonadal dysgenesis XX and two were carriers of Turner Syndrome. [2]

The gonadoblastomas are more frequently observed in the second decade of life, unless the cancer occurs in cryptorchid testes. In one reported case, a dysgerminoma was diagnosed shortly after birth. About 20% arise in dysgenetic gonads and 18% in dysgenetics cryptorchid testes and in 60% of cases, the original structure of the gonad is hidden by the tumor and therefore undetermined. [2]

A gonadoblastoma can synthesize estrogen or testosterone, which may account for the feminization or even for the masculinization, that is sometimes present in XY gonadal dysgenesis. [4]

The gonadoblastomas may be associated with disgerminomas (50%) and other malignant germ cell elements (10%) [3], and the clinical prognosis is associated with the presence or absence of these elements. Pure gonadoblastomas not metastasize, unlike disgerminomas, which nevertheless respond well to radiotherapy, with infrequent and late recurrence. On the other hand, embryonal carcinoma, endodermal tumors of the sinus, choriocarcinoma and immature teratomas are highly malignant and often lethal if not treated with multiple drug therapy. [12]

The occurrence of gonadal tumors (gonadoblastoma or dysgerminoma) in XY gonadal dysgenesis patients is about 30%, based on retrospective analysis. The prevalence in familial cases appears to be greater. In 62 familial cases, 38 subjects (58%) had gonadal tumors, primarily gonadoblastomas or disgerminomas. Verp and Simpson [2] found eleven cases of gonadal tumors in 45 non-familial cases (24%). The disgerminomas are the only malignant tumors germ cell with a substantial incidence of bilaterality, which occurs in 15% of cases. [12]

Even though gonadoblastoma is the most feared in situ malignancy of the dysgenetic gonads, other nontumoral androgen-producing lesions may be related to the presence of hidden or overt Y-chromosome sequences. Temporal exposure of a dysgenetic gonad presenting Y-chromosome–specific sequences could lead to a clinical picture of hyperandrogenism, because of accumulated modifications in the gonadal microenvironment. However, no correlation was found concerning hyperandrogenism and the presence of Y-chromosome sequences in patients presenting disgenetic gonads. [11]

These findings are consistent with the clinical observation that patients with a translocation of the *SRY* gene to an X chromosome or an autosome, resulting in 46,XX males, have no increased risk for this type of cancer and thereby do not exclude the possible role of *SRY* in the development of these malignancies.

It can also be noted that during embryonic development, the XY germ cells divide more rapidly than XX. Thus, XY germ cells, originally programmed to run at a place with milder temperature (*scrotum*) and under a low metabolic rate, must respond to this intra-abdominal position with an abnormal increase in metabolic rate and thus with propensity to neoplastic transformation.

Elevated levels of gonadotropins by themselves are not only likely oncogenic as observed low rates of neoplasia in individuals 45 X. [11]

In addition, Bianco et al. [10] investigated the presence of Y-chromosome mosaicism (*SRY*, *TSPY* and *DYZE*) in 87 TS patients by means of PCR, along with its association with the development of gonadal tumors and/or nontumoral androgen-producing lesions. The data revealed hidden Y-chromosome mosaicism in 18.5% of the patients. The *SRY* sequence was detected in all of these patients, while 4.6% of them presented the *DYZ3* repeat region and 4.6% of them presented the *TSPY* gene. Eleven of the patients with Y-positive sequences agreed to undergo prophylactic surgery. In two cases, bilateral gonadoblastoma was found and, in another case, histopathological analysis on the gonads revealed hilus cell hyperplasia. In a further case, hilus cell hyperplasia and stromal luteoma were found. These authors concluded that a systematic search for hidden Y-chromosome mosaicism, especially for the *SRY* gene, in Turner syndrome patients, was justified because of the possibility of preventing gonadal lesions.

Klinefelter Syndrome; Occurrence of Mediastinal Type II GCTs

Klinefelter syndrome patients (47,XXY), a variant of sex chromosomal DSD, have no increased risk of type II GCTs of the testis, but rather of the mediastinum. [4] The absence of gonadal (testicular) GCTs in these patients is likely due to induction of apoptosis of germ cells related to an improper microenvironment. [4, 11] The resulting pituitary/gonadal overstimulation may play a role in the formation of the mediastinal tumour. Indications of apoptosis of gonadal germ cells have also been reported in the ovary of Turner syndrome patients (45,X), another variant of sex chromosomal DSD, as well as patients with complete androgen insensitivity, a variant of 46,XY DSD.

Parameters Related to Gonadal Type II GCT Risk in DSD

DSD patients with hypervirilisation (various forms of 46,XX DSD with androgen excess in the new classification) [4] do not have an increased risk for GCTs compared with the general population. However, this is completely different for DSD patients with either hypovirilisation or gonadal dysgenesis. These can in fact be part of all three categories in the new classification: sex chromosomal DSD, 46, XY DSD and 46, XX DSD. Several reviews on this topic have been published recently. [4]

In summary, only the DSD patients with hypovirilisation or gonadal dysgenesis may have an increased risk for development of type II GCTs, although in a highly heterogeneous pattern. This is found to be related to several specific parameters. In summary, almost all these patients are at risk for gonadal GCTs. [4]

Gonadal Localization

The anatomical position of the gonad is an informative predictive parameter for development of gonadal type II GCTs. This is in line with the fact that cryptorchidism is one of the strongest risk factors for type II GCTs of the testis in the general (Caucasian) population. [4] Indeed, within DSD patients, the risk for tumour development is higher within the same patient category when the gonad is abdominal rather than scrotal. This is only the case if the other requirements for malignant transformation of germ cells are fulfilled, including the presence of the so-called GBY region. Interestingly, it has been demonstrated that a seminomatous histology of the tumour is more frequently found in intra-abdominal testes than in testes localized in the scrotum. This likely also explains the preferential occurrence of dysgerminomas in the ovary as well as dysgenetic gonad, which are abdominally located. In view of these observations, it comes as no surprise that seminoma of the testis and dysgerminoma of the dysgenetic gonad/ovary are similar regarding morphology, immunohistochemical characteristics, chromosomal constitution as well as gene expression profile. Precursor lesion depending on gonadal virilisation status as indicated above, the precursor of type II gonadal GCTs can be either CIS/IGCNU or GB, or a combination of both. [4,7] This is in fact found to be related to the level of testicularisation of the gonad: CIS in the testis and GB in the dysgenetic (undifferentiated) gonad, or a mixture of both. This can be well demonstrated by the use of immunohistochemistry for *SOX9* (read-out of *SRY* function and Sertoli cell differentiation) and *FOXL2* (granulose cell differentiation). These results indicate that CIS/ IGCNU and GB are part of a histological continuum, as originally proposed, in which the development into either Sertoli–or granulosa–cell direction determines the histological context of the premalignant cells. The precursor lesion of GB has been identified, being UGT, allowing a better histological description of the gonadal tissue available, either a biopsy or gonadectomy specimen. Again, PGC/gonocyte-like premalignant germ cells are present in these UGT lesions, being *OCT3/4* (*AP* and *KIT*) positive. In addition, the stromal cells show expression of predominantly *FOXL2* compared to *SOX9*. [4, 7]

Involvement of the Y Chromosome

The highest incidence of tumors in patients with gonadal dysgenesis and the presence of Y chromosome may be related to two factors: (1) undifferentiated gonadal tissue would, by its own nature, prone to neoplastic transformation, regardless of the mechanism of genetic origin of gonadal dysgenesis, (2) the gene that produces gonadal dysgenesis not only cause the absence of germ cells, but also confer malignant properties namely, hypoplasia and gonadal neoplasia were related phenomena. [4]

The increased prevalence of cancer may arise from the presence of undifferentiated XY gonadal tissue in an environment abnormal (intraabdominal). This hypothesis is reinforced by observations that the prevalence of gonadal neoplasms are also increased in intra-abdominal 45, X/46, XY dysgenetic gonads and also by the finding of tumors in cryptorchid testes. [2]

The increased risk of developing gonadoblastoma in patients with gonadal dysgenetic and material derived from the presence of Y chromosome in their chromosome constitution is well established and caused Page to postulate in 1987 [13] the existence of a gene (GBY) on the Y chromosome with this function. Page suggested that the location of GBY was near the centromere or on the long arm of Y chromosome, therefore different from the location of *SRY*.

In 1995, Tsuchiya et al. [4] used several Y chromosome specific probes to study cases of sex reversal, gonadoblastoma and the presence of Y chromosome in karyotype. According to the authors, the gene GBY would be located in a small region near the centromere, estimated at approximately 1-2Mb. The analysis indicated that both *TSPY* (Ypter-p11.2) as *YRRM* (Y-chromosome RNA Recognition Motif - Yq11) were present in all cases.

Despite these results, *YRRM* or *TSPY* were not directly involved in the etiology of gonadoblastoma, it is also believed that the GBY critical region may be just one or even multiple loci on Y chromosome. [4]

Our findings do not support the suggestion that the presence of TSPY gene is a triggering factor causing the neoplastic process in dysgenetic gonads as has been suggested in a number of previous studies. [3, 4, 6] SRY is expressed before *TSPY* in the sex differentiation cascade, reinforcing the role of this gene in the abnormal microenvironment of dysgenetic gonads, as the main determinant of neoplastic progression, providing the cell with equipment to survive and proliferate. [9, 11]

The mutant gene that determines the XY PGD, for example *SRY* could give directly the tendency to neoplastic transformation. This hypothesis is based on the early age of onset of cancer and the relatively high frequency of bilaterality, tumor characteristics associated with gene mutations. It was observed that fibroblasts from patients with XY PGD, but not those with lineage containing mosaicism 45, X, are most susceptible to transformation after exposure to SV40 (simian virus papoma). [14] Although the mechanism is unknown, there are at least three current hypotheses: [14]

(1) The mutation which determines XY PGD may also lead to the emergence of aneuploid lines of germ cells;
(2) The mutant gene could alter the cell surface antigens in embryonic cells. Bennett et al. made several observations relevant to this point in mice;
(3) The mutated gene may be a tumor suppressor, following the model proposed by Knudson et al. This hypothesis can be supported by the fact that virtually all gonadoblastomas occur in patients 45, X/46, XY or XY gonadal dysgenesis and is rarely observed in 46, XX subjects and only once was detected in a patient with ataxia telangiectasia, a disorder characterized by chromosome instability.

Complete gonadal dysgenesis (CGD) and subtypes of 46XY DSD with abdominal gonads carry the highest risk and tumours develop in 35% of these patients. Female 46XY patients within this subgroup of DSD have small, often streak-like gonads with absent or minimal function. They must balance their tumour risk mainly against that of unnecessary surgery. Given the low risk in some subgroups, the practice of early gonadectomy regardless of diagnosis is intensely debated. At a microscopic level, the borderline between a neoplasia and a delay of maturation is hard to define. Imaging of the gonads by US or MRI is difficult because of the small size and the variable localisation. Some of these gonads are very mobile, making the serial imaging by US challenging. For these reasons, early gonadectomy is usually advised for all patients. [12]

References

[1] Hughes JF, Rozen S. Genomics and Genetics of Human and primate Y Chromosomes. *Annu. Rev.Genomics Hum. Genet.* 2012: p. 3.1-3.26.

[2] Lipay MVN, Bianco B, Verreschi ITN. Disgenesias Gonadais e Tumores: Aspectos Genéticos e Clínicos. Arq Bras Endocrinol Metabol. 2005: p. 60-70.
[3] Looijenga LHJ, Hersmus R, Cools M, Drop SLS, Wolffenbuttel KP. Tumor risk in disorders of sex development (DSD). *Best Practice and Research Clinical Endocrinology and Metabolism.* 2007: p. 480-495.
[4] Looijenga LHJ, Hersmus R, de Leeuw BHCGM, Stoop H, Cools M, Oosterhuis JW, et al. Gonadal tumours and DSD. *Best Practice and Research Clinical Endocrinology and Metabolism.* 2010: p. 291-310.
[5] Franco HL, Yao HHC. Sex and Hedgehog: roles of genes in the hedgehog signaling patway in mammalian sexual differentiation. *Chromosome Research.* 2012: p. 247-258.
[6] Looijenga L. Genetic basis of testicular tumors. *Endocrine Abstracts.* 2007: p. S23.4.
[7] Cools M, Looijenga LHJ, Wolffenbuttel KP, Drop SLS. Disorders of sex development: update on the genetic background, terminology and risk for the development of germ cell tumors. *World J. Pediatr.* 2009: p. 93-102.
[8] Bianco B, Lipay MV, Melaragno MI, Guedes AD, Verreschi IT. Detection of hidden Y mosaicism in Turner's syndrome: importance in the prevention of gonadoblastoma. *J. Pediatr. Endocrinol. Metab.* 2006: p. 1113-7.
[9] Bianco B, Lipay MVN, Guedes AD, Verreschi ITN. Clinical implications of the detection of Y-chromosome mosaicism in Turner's syndrome: report of 3 cases. *Fertility and Sterility.* 2008: p. e.17-e.20.
[10] Bianco B, Lipay M, Guedes A, Oliveira K, Verreschi I. SRY gene increases the risk of developing gonadoblastoma and/or nontumoral gonadal lesions in Turner syndrome. *International Journal of Ginecological Pathology.* 2009: p. 197-202.
[11] Bianco B, Oliveira KC, Guedes AD, Barbosa C, Lipay MVN, Verreschi ITN. OCT4 gonadal gene expression related to the presence of Y-chromosome sequences in Turner syndrome. *Fertility and Sterility.* 2010: p. 2347-2349.
[12] Wünsch L, Holterhus PM, Wessel L, Hiort O. Patients with disorders of sex development (DSD) at risk of gonadal tumour development: management based on laparoscopic biopsy and molecular diagnosis. *BJU International.* 2012: p. 1464-410.

[13] Page DC, Mosher R, Simpson EM, Fisher EM, Mardon G, Pollack J, et al. The sex-determining region of the human Y chromosome encodes a finger protein. *Cell*. 1987: p. 1091-104.
[14] Oliveira RMR, Verreschi ITN, Lipay MVN, Eça LP, Guedes AD, Bianco B. Y chromosome in Turner syndrome: review of the literature. *Sao Paulo Medical Journal*. 2009: p. 373-378.

In: Sex Chromosomes: New Research ISBN: 978-1-62417-143-7
Editors: M. D'Aquino and V. Stallone © 2013 Nova Science Publishers, Inc.

Chapter V

Deletion of Amelogenin Y-Locus: State of the Art in Gender Determination

Luciana Caenazzo and Pamela Tozzo
Department of Molecular Medicine, University of Padua, Padova, Italy

Abstract

Accurate gender determination is widely used and it is crucial in many scientific disciplines, especially in profiling for DNA databasing, forensic casework (e.g., identifying the gender of biological material in stains of unknown origin), analysis of archeological specimens, preimplantation/prenatal diagnosis and post-natal diagnosis (e.g., X-linked diseases or children with ambiguous genitals). Today, molecular techniques, also based on length variation in the X–Y homologous amelogenin gene (AMELX and AMELY), are used for sex determination. In humans, the amelogenin gene is a single copy gene located on Xp22.1–Xp22.3 and Yp11.2 and it is sufficiently conserved, so the simultaneous detection of the X and Y alleles using polymerase chain reaction can lead to gender determination. There is a size difference of 6 bp between the X and the Y genes in the most widely used PCR primer set. The presence of two amplified products indicates a male genotype, while a single amplicon implies a female genotype. Several studies, published since 1998, have shown that normal males may be typed as females with this test because the amelogenin gender test may not always be concordant with true male gender: AMELY deletions may result in no amplification product and normal males being typed as female with the test (negative male). To date literature data have supported that the null allele is the result of a larger deletion on the short arm of the Y chromosome and that this occurs in different percentages in different population groups. Considering the consequences of the result obtained using only the amelogenin marker and the potential related interpretation difficulties, the gender misinterpretation may be troublesome in some cases, both in clinical practice and forensic caseworks. Different strategies have been proposed to solve this misinterpretation, such as the use of additional markers to resolve the possible occurrence of AMEY deletion. In this paper we propose a review of the incidence in failures of gender testing among different populations and the different strategies proposed in literature in case of doubt regarding the presence of deleted AME in the DNA profile.

Introduction

The human amelogenin gene, sequenced by Nakahori et al. [1991], which is highly conserved in primates [Bayley et al., 1992], is located on both the X and Y chromosome, as single copies, in homologous regions and it is widely used in different fields. The human AMELX-gene has a size of 2872 bp and is located on the p22 region of the X-chromosome, while the human AMELY-gene has a size of 3272 bp and is located on the 11p12.2 region of the Y-chromosome. Amelogenin is a gene that codes for a matrix protein forming tooth enamel, in which it represents 90% of the organic content [Richard et al., 2007] and in males AMELY is expressed at a low level. AMELX has an important role in determining the development of normal enamel structure, composition and thickness, and several mutations at this locus lead to X-linked amelogenesis imperfecta [Hart et al., 2002].

There is a difference in an intronic part of amelogenin gene between X-linked amelogenin (AMELX) and Y-linked amelogenin (AMELY). In particular, PCR products generated from AMELX and AMELY chromosome can be discriminated one from the other using primers flanking a 6 bp deletion in the first intron of the X chromosome. Sequence differences between the X and Y homologues of the amelogenin gene have been used to differentiate males from females with ambiguous phenotype or to establish the gender in biological material analysis for different purposes. Since both X- and Y-specific fragments can be amplified in a single reaction, amplification of the amelogenin gene offers the advantage of having an internal positive control represented by the X chromosome homologous fragment, which should always be present. The two most commonly used amelogenin primer sets span a 6 base pair (bp) deletion on the X chromosome and generate fragments of 106/112 bp or 212/218 bp for X/Y products, respectively [Sullivan et al., 1993; Mannucci et al., 1994]. Several companies manufacture amelogenin primer sets for sex identification, as well as multiplex short tandem repeat (STR) kits, contain primers specific for the amelogenin gene which allows for individual as well as gender identification.

The most widely used application of STR analysis is in forensics. However, DNA typing applications in other fields are gaining in popularity and include testing to monitor the follow-up after allogenic bone marrow transplantation [Ghaffari et al., 2008], evaluating the origin of tumors inadvertently transmitted by solid organ transplantation [Shadrach et al., 2004], analysis of archeological specimens [Gibbon et al. 2009], preimplantation/prenatal diagnosis and post-natal diagnosis (e.g., X-linked diseases or children with ambiguous genitals) [Caenazzo et al., 1997; Bianchi et al., 2004; Zhu et al., 2005].

In forensics, the use of multiplex-PCR systems with additional amelogenin detections leads to sex determination of traces. It is useful, in particular, in sexual assault cases, to distinguish between the victim and the perpetrator's evidence, in case of sex determination of remains in mass disasters or investigations regarding missing persons. It can also help to resolve sample mix-ups. A particular aspect is the application of amelogenin-based sex determination in ancient DNA studies. This approach provides a solution in case of ancient biological material lacking clear morphological diagnostic features, for example, in case of fragmentary or juvenile skeletal remains. In archeological fields gender determination is important in assessing sex-specific demographic data (for example age and stature), to better understand the gender and sex specific roles in old societies. However, it must be stated that the traditional and molecular methods of sex identification complement each other, and where one fails the other may succeed [Gibbon et al. 2009]. The importance of sex discrimination may arise when facing, in clinical practice, different situations. Monitoring the engraftment of the donor cells, after allogenic peripheral blood stem cell transplantation, may be important for the early diagnosis of graft failure. In some cases, detection of mixed chimerism can be predictive of imminent relapse. After allogenic BMT (Bone Marrow Transplantation), it is of interest to monitor the recipient's circulating cell populations in order to assess the haematological changes resulting from the transfusion of donor marrow. Many genetic markers are available to detect chimerism and they vary with respect to sensitivity and effectiveness. In the case of sex-mismatched donor recipient pairs, information about the ratio between donor and recipient can be efficiently obtained using PCR-based amplification of amelogenin homologous sequences; in fact amelogenin gene amplification allows detection of both male and female cells by a single-step PCR reaction simultaneously. The application of this assessment can be used not only for PCR-based sex determination but also for analyzing relative quantification of mixed chimerism and for observing the kinetics of engraftment. A particular situation which has to be highlighted, involving both forensic and clinical aspects, is that after successful allogenic bone marrow transplantation in sex-mismatched donor recipient pairs, the amelogenin-based sex determined in the blood samples (hematopoietic cell lines) of the recipient is the same of the donor, but it is different from the sex determined in the DNA obtained from the recipient's structural cells [von Wurmb-Schwark et al., 2007]. The determination of sex chromosomes through the PCR amplification of amelogenin gene can be useful in prenatal diagnosis of congenital adrenal hyperplasia or X-linked disorders, such as Duchenne muscular dystrophy, Wiscott-Aldrich syndrome, Hunter's syndrome, or in diagnosis and management of patients with intersex (testicular feminization syndrome, male pseudohermaphroditism, true hermaphroditism) [Chowdhuri et al., 1998]. In particular, Zhu and collaborators in 2005 studied the possibility to use the 6 bp difference between AMELX and AMELY for non-invasive prenatal fetal gender or diagnosis of paternally inherited disorders, since the presence of fetal DNA in maternal plasma and serum has offered new approaches to non-invasive prenatal diagnosis [Zhu et al., in 2005]. One potential clinical application in the field of prenatal diagnosis is to determine which pregnant women should receive treatments for a potential fetus with congenital adrenal hyperplasia [Bianchi, 2004].

Pitfalls in Gender Determination Typing Amelogenin Gene

AMELY Drop-out

Several studies in literature to date have reported mutations in the AMELY homologue gene which can cause typing of males as females with noteworthy consequences if used, for example, in cases of criminal investigation (forensic/rape cases), in identifying human remains from mass disasters or for gender identification in the setting of prenatal diagnosis of X-linked recessive diseases as mentioned above.

Santos et al. for the first time reported that the amelogenin-based sex test incorrectly types some males as females because they lack the AMELY as a result of a deletion polymorphism. They considered 350 individuals coming from different countries and reported two cases of amelogenin-based sex test failure: they both came from Sri Lanka (0.6% frequency of sex test failures due to deletion polymorphisms in the sample). The same Authors observed a deletion frequency of 8% within their Sri Lankan population sample (n=24) suggesting that in some populations the frequency of failure might be higher; they proposed as the mutation mechanism a recombination between the TSPYA and TSPYB loci [Santos et al., 1998]. Other cases of AMELY mutations have been reported [Hart et al., 2000; Roffey et al., 2000; Brinkman, 2002] and some Authors have argued that the AMELY null result might be due to a point mutation within the primer binding site region rather than a deletion of the AMELY sequence [Roffey et al., 2000; Henke et al., 2001].

Thangaraj et al. investigated a total of 270 Indian male samples finding that 5 individuals showed deletion polymorphisms of about 1 MB encompassing the AMELY locus on Yp, defined through Southern hybridization, with an observed amplification failure frequency of 1.85% [Thangaraj et al., 2002]. Steinlechner and collaborators reported that in a population sample of 29432 phenotypic males stored in the Austrian National DNA database, 6 individuals lacked the AMELY PCR amplification, resulting in wrong gender determination with observed frequency of amelogenin-based sex test failure of 0.018%. In this study the sex could be correctly determined by typing Y-STR loci in five cases and in one case by typing SRY. [Steinlechner et al., 2002]. Chang et al. in 2003 described a 3.6% failure rate of the amelogenin-based sex test in an Indian population group from Malaysia (population sample of 338 males, 113 Malays, 113 Chinese and 112 Indians) and they found the drop-out of both AMELY and MSY1 minisatellite loci, showing that the deletion spanned a length in the order of probably several Kb [Chang et al., 2003]. A bigger Malaysian population group (n=980, 334 Malays, 331 Chinese and 315 Indians) was studied in 2007, showing that both the Indians and Malays exhibited amelogenin-null frequency of 3.2% and 0.6% respectively. The two studied identified a similar deletion region on the Yp 11.2 band of at least 1.13 Mb, encompassing the AMELY, MSY1 minisatellite and DYS458 locus. The haplogroup results for the Indian nulls indicated an ancestral J2e lineage [Chang et al., 2007].

As failure in gender determination was found to be particularly high in males originating from India, Kashyap et al. analyzed the amelogenin typing results of 4257 males originating from different regions of India and included in the DNA databasing project. Among this individuals, 10 confirmed males showed a drop-out of the 112 bp AMELY gene and the overall failure rate was 0.23%. They were tested with alternate primers pairs encompassing the previously amplified region and they failed amplification. Additional analysis with male-specific SRY locus, with 4 Y-specific STR polymorphisms and Y-SNPs were performed and the Authors inferred that the deletion spanned a region downstream of the reverse primer-binding site of commercially available amelogenin primer sets [Kashyap et al., 2006].

In 2004, the Israel Defence Force reported the failure of an amelogenin-based sex test on a phenotypically normal male soldier [Michael et al., 2004].

Lattanzi et al. described an interstitial deletion of the Y short arm encompassing the AMELY locus in two cases of unrelated individuals: one case was identified during the screening for Y microdeletions performed on a sample of 493 infertile males while the second one was found among 13000 amniotic liquid samples from male fetus pregnancies tested by quantitative fluorescence-polymerase chain reaction (QF-PCR) and cytogenetic analysis for prenatal diagnosis. In order to estimate the extent of the deletion on Yp the researchers performed a pulsed-field gel electrophoresis (PFGE), followed by fluorescence in situ hybridization (FISH) and sequence-tagged site (STS) marker analysis and the deletion size was about 2.5 Mb. An intact SRY locus was present in both individuals and, considering that the two carriers of the deletion had different Y-STR haplotypes, it was supposed that the mutation has occurred independently or that there has been an old single mutational event [Lattanzi et al., 2005].

In Australia the frequency of AMELY amplification drop-out reported by Mitchell et al. was low (0.02%) in a population sample of 109,000 males. The samples of 5 AMELY-null males (2 of Indian origin, one Italian and two of South-Asian) were typed for eight sequence tagged sites (STS) located on Yp using PCR and gel electrophoresis and also for eleven Y-specific STR to study haplotypes for phylogenetic analysis. In the five samples two different sized deletions were identified (ranging between 304-731 and 712-1001 Kb) [Mitchell et al., 2006].

In a sample population of 77 males from Kathmandu, Nepal, 5 null AMELY individuals were found (6.49%). In this case the deletion size was estimated to be of about 2.3 Mb, through a battery of male-specific SNPs, STRs, STSs and minisatellite; furthermore, considering the Y-haplogroup analysis performed, all five individuals were belonging to the same lineage (J2b2-M241) [Cadenas et al., 2007]. Literature data suggest a concentration of AMELY null individuals in the Indian subcontinent, possibly as a result of common ancestry.

Jobling et al. analyzed a total of 45 AMELY-null males from different origin (among these 32 have already been reported in Literature by other researchers) and studied a combination of STSs deletion mapping, binary-marker and Y-haplotyping, and TSPY copy number estimation to understand the structural basis of the deletions involved. The Authors reported four different deletion classes, ranging from 2.5 Mb and 4.0 Mb, due to a total of ten independent events [Jobling et al., 2007].

Two cases of AMELY deletion have been reported in the North-east Italian population: in the first case an alleged father-son pair were erroneously typed as females, in the second case the AMELY deletion was found on a sample of amniotic fluid collected during prenatal diagnosis of a male fetus pregnancy. The Authors suggested a deletion range of 3.35-3.87 Mb in the first case and 1.51-2.58 Mb in the second case respectively. Furthermore, the two cases showed different haplotypes and different deletion breakpoints [Turrina et al., 2011]. In a Japanese casework involving two dead brothers and two of their male relatives, all the four males were lacking the amelogenin Y homologous. Investigation using Y-specific markers showed a deletion of about 2.56 Mb in the Yp11.2 region [Kumagai et al., 2008]. Thereafter, the same research group found another case of a Japanese AMELY-null male and they performed, in both cases, the high resolution STS mapping and the Y haplogroup analysis. They argued a deletion mechanism of non-homologous end-joining and that the two deletion events had occurred independently [Kumagai et al., 2010]. Another case of amelogenin-null male was reported in Japan and the sizes of the identified deletions were approximately of 2.51 Mb, 25 kb and 834 b and the Y-STR haplotype was different from those previously reported in literature [Takayama et al., 2009]. Considering the different deletion distribution among the populations reported in scientific literature we can conclude that observed frequencies of the amelogenin sex testing failures show population-specific difference.

Other Methods for Gender Determination

In order to solve the problem related with null AMELY males, different approaches have been settled for gender determination, especially in forensics and prenatal diagnosis. Haas-Rocholz and Weiler investigated the size of flanking sequences of homologous regions of the AMELX and the AMELY gene for possible primers producing PCR fragments smaller than those described by Sullivan, and they suggested primers AMELU1 and AMELD1, resulting in a 80 bp X-chromosome specific and a 83 bp Y-chromosome specific fragment [Haas-Rocholz and Weiler, 1997].

However, for the reasons mention above, also with these shorter PCR products in the amelogenin-based sex test the possibility of incorrect gender determination remains.

Some Studies have investigated the use of genetic markers lying in the sex-determination region Y (SRY) of the Y chromosome as additional singleplex PCR first and then in combination with AMEL primers, but these procedures were more lengthy and led to consuming more time and a greater sample amount [Skaletsky et al., 2003; Thangaraji et al., 2002; Jobling et a., 2007].

Nevertheless, this method, if used as a singleplex of SRY, can not accurately indicate a female genotype because the amplicon may be absent due to degraded DNA in the examined specimen.

On the other hand, if SRY is co-amplified with AMEL, it helps the detection of AMELY-null samples, so some different Authors have proposed in literature different method for associate a Y-specific marker to AMEL.

SRY is thought to direct the sex-determination pathway towards male development. It has been demonstrated [Drobnic, 2006] and validated [Kastelic et al., 2009] that the SRY gene test for gender determination can be incorporated into other STR analyses with commercial kits which also contain AMEL. The advantage of this assay is that the PCR product of this novel marker residing in the SRY gene is 96 bp long, thus providing feasible gender determination when typing degraded forensic samples. Furthermore, the SRY amplification product does not migrate with any of the AMEL or STR alleles in the multiplex STR kits because of its short length, so it can be easily used as a singleplex or included in multiplex kits.

Giuliodori et al. have developed a method for the identification of AMELY-null samples, based on a small polyacrylamide-gel electrophoresis of a duplex PCR product of a new marker residing in the SRY gene, which results in a 197 bp long PCR product, in combination with primers for AMEL. This method can be applied, as an additional test, in case of doubt regarding the presence of deleted AME in the DNA profile. This approach was based on the direct visualization of the small polyacrylamide gel of the bands corresponding to the two respective amplified fragments. In normal conditions, the female shows a band of 106 bp (AMELX) with no band corresponding to SRY while the male shows three bands respectively, 106 bp and 112 bp for AMELX and AMELY respectively, and 197 bp for SRY. In case of AMELY drop-out, the male shows two bands: only 106 bp for AMELX and 197 bp for SRY. This method is sensitive, reliable and it successfully types DNA derived from forensic samples, and it can be used to identify males with the amelogenin deletion in stains analyzed for forensic caseworks and also for gender diagnosis in particular cases [Giuliodori et al., 2011].

A completely different approach is the one proposed by Andréasson and Allen [2003], in which the sex determination test is performed with a real-time PCR assay, based on melting curve analysis, while an externally standardized kinetic analysis allows quantification of the nuclear DNA copy number in the sample.

Morikawa et al. have developed a method for sex determination using a multiplex amplification of SRY, STS (steroid sulfatase) and amelogenin gene regions and their homologous sequences. For this method a detection limit of 63 pg of genomic DNA was demonstrated, and the male DNA component could be detected from mixed samples with a male:female ratio as low as 1:10. [Morikawa et al., 2011].

Furthermore, the pentanucleotide microsatellite DXYS156 maps to the pseudoautosomal region of both sex chromosomes and can be used for sex determination [Chen et al., 2010]. It is a multiallelic STR with geographic-specific allelic distribution, helping not only the determination of sex but also of the probable geographical origin of an individual. The Y-specific alleles can be distinguished from the X-specific alleles because of an adenine insertion in the repeat units of the STR [Mukerjee et al., 2011].

While the AMELY deletion may lead to incorrect determination of sex, the AMELX deletion doesn't affect amelogenin-based sex test: in fact, in case of a true female subject the AMELX deletion in one X chromosome remains undetected and in case of a true male subject there will be the only AMELY fragment amplification suggesting the failure of AMELX amplification. Obviously the PCR drop-out of both X-homologues amelogenin loci in a true female subject clearly suggests that there have been some troubles in gender determination by using amelogenin gene. However, if used quantitatively to determine certain sex chromosome aneuploidies such as XXY, the X homologue PCR drop-out could lead to incorrect determinations of X copies number with subsequent incorrect characterization of sex chromosome abnormalities.

The PCR drop-out of the X-homologue of the amelogenin gene has been rarely reported in literature, often as a consequence of point mutations in PCR primers binding sites [Shadrach et al., 2004; Alves et al., 2004]. Caratti et al., testing over 43000 individuals through routine QF-PCR (Quantitative Fluorescent Polymerase Chain Reaction), observed a single Caucasian male originating from northeast Italy lacking amplification of AMELX with normal genotypes at pseudoautosomal and X-chromosomal STR loci [Caratti et al., 2009]. In this case the cause of the AMELX drop-out was identified in a point mutation in the annealing region of primers included in the amplification kit rather than a deletion. The mutation described by Caratti et al. was identical to that reported by Shadrach et al. in a Caucasian (population sample of 327 individuals of unspecified ethnic origin from the United States of America) and by Maciejewska and Pawlowski in a Caucasian male (population sample of 5534 Polish males) [Maciejewska and Pawlowski, 2009].

Conclusion

Genotyping the X-Y homologous amelogenin gene segment for gender identification is widely used in biological material analysis for different purposes as forensic casework, archeological specimens, preimplantation and prenatal diagnoses and detection of mixed chimerism.

Since both X- and Y-specific fragments can be amplified in a single reaction, amplification of the amelogenin gene offers the advantage of having an internal positive control represented by the X chromosome homologous fragment which should always be present.

However, the fallibility of the amelogenin-based sex test raises concern. The consequences of erroneous gender determination may be noteworthy in different fields. The observed amelogenin sex test failure rates in different populations should be considered and an increasing contribution from population-studies in this field is desirable. It would be important to know the failure rate among different ethnic groups, even those which have not been studied to date. The pitfalls in amelogenin-based sex determination may be overcome by adequate and common methodological approaches that involve co-amplification with other Y chromosome markers.

References

Alves C, Coelho M, Rocha J, Amorim A. 2006. The Amelogenin locus displays a high frequency of X homologue failures in Sao Tome Island (West Africa). In Progress in Forensic Genetics 11, Amorim A, Corte-Real F, Morling N (eds). Elsevier Science: Amsterdam; 271-3.

Andréasson H, Allen M. Rapid quantification and sex determination of forensic evidence materials. *J. Forensic Sci.* 2003 Nov;48(6):1280-7.

Bayley DMD, Affra NA, Fergusons-Smith M. The X–Y homologous gene amelogenin maps to the short arms of both the X and the Y chromosomes and is highly conserved in primates. *Genomics.* 1992;14:203-5.

Bianchi DW. Circulating fetal DNA: its origin and diagnostic potential-a review. *Placenta.* 2004 Apr;25 Suppl A:S93-S101.

Brinkmann B. Is the amelogenin sex test valid? *Int. J. Legal Med.* (2002) 116:63.

Cadenas AM, Regueiro M, Gayden T, Singh N, Zhivotovsky LA, Underhill PA, Herrera RJ. Male amelogenin dropouts: phylogenetic context, origins and implications. *Forensic. Sci. Int.* 2007 Mar 2;166(2-3):155-63.

Caenazzo L, Ponzano E, Greggio NA, Cortivo P. Prenatal sexing and sex determination in infants with ambiguous genitalia by polymerase chain reaction. *Genet. Test.* 1997-1998;1(4):289-91.

Caratti S, Voglino G, Cirigliano V, Ghidini A, Taulli R, Torre C, Robino C. Amplification failure of the amelogenin gene (AMELX) caused by a primer binding site mutation. *Prenat. Diagn.* 2009 Dec;29(12):1180-2.

Chang YM, Burgoyne LA, Both K. Higher failures of amelogenin sex test in an Indian population group. *J. Forensic Sci.* 2003 Nov;48(6):1309-13.

Chang YM, Perumal R, Keat PY, Yong RY, Kuehn DL, Burgoyne L. A distinct Y-STR haplotype for Amelogenin negative males characterized by a large Y(p)11.2 (DYS458-MSY1-AMEL-Y) deletion. *Forensic Sci. Int.* 2007 Mar;166(2-3):115-20.

Chen H, Lowther W, Avramopoulos D, Antonarakis SE. Homologous loci DXYS156X and DXYS156Y contain a polymorphic pentanucleotide repeat (TAAAA)n and map to human X and Y chromosomes. *Hum. Mutat.* 1994;4(3):208-11.

Chowdhury MR, Mathur R, Verma IC. Utility of XY-amelogenin gene primers for detection of sex chromosomes. *Indian J. Med. Res.* 1998 Apr;107:182-6.

Drobnič K. A new primer set in a SRY gene for sex identification. 2006. In Progress in Forensic Genetics 11, Amorim A, Corte-Real F, Morling N (eds). Elsevier Science: Amsterdam; 268-70.

Ghaffari SH, Chahardouli B, Gavamzadeh A, Alimoghaddam K. Evaluation of hematopoietic chimerism following allogeneic peripheral blood stem cell transplantation with amelogenin marker. *Arch. Iran Med.* 2008 Jan;11(1):35-41.

Gibbon V, Paximadis M, Strkalj G, Ruff P, Penny C. Novel methods of molecular sex identification from skeletal tissue using the amelogenin gene. *Forensic Sci. Int. Genet.* 2009 Mar;3(2):74-9.

Giuliodori A, Corato S, Ponzano E, Rodriguez D, Caenazzo L. Rapid analysis for confirmation of amelogenin negative males characterized by a Yp11.2 deletion. *Forensic Sci. Int. Genet. Supplement Series* 3 2011:e285-e286.

Haas-Rochholz H, Weiler G. Additional primer sets for an amelogenin gene PCR-based DNA-sex test. *Int. J. Legal Med.* 1997;110(6):312-5.

Hart PS, Vlaservich AC, Hart TC, Wright JT. Polymorphism (g2035C>T) in the amelogenin gene. *Hum. Mutat.* 2000 Mar;15(3):298.

Hart PS, Hart TC, Simmer JP, Wright J. A nomenclature for Xlinked amelogenesis imperfecta. *Arch. Oral Biol.* 2002;47: 255-60.

Henke J, Henke L, Chatthopadhyay P, Kayser M, Dülmer M, Cleef S, Pöche H, Felske-Zech H. Application of Y-chromosomal STR haplotypes to forensic genetics. *Croat. Med. J.* 2001 Jun;42(3):292-7.

Jobling MA, Lo IC, Turner DJ, Bowden GR, Lee AC, Xue Y, Carvalho-Silva D, Hurles ME, Adams SM, Chang YM, Kraaijenbrink T, Henke J, Guanti G, McKeown B, van Oorschot RA, Mitchell RJ, de Knijff P, Tyler-Smith C, Parkin EJ. Structural variation on the short arm of the human Y chromosome: recurrent multigene deletions encompassing Amelogenin Y. *Hum. Mol. Genet.* 2007 Feb;16(3):307-16.

Kashyap VK, Sahoo S, Sitalaximi T, Trivedi R. Deletions in the Y-derived amelogenin gene fragment in the Indian population. *BMC Med. Genet.* 2006 Apr;7:37.

Kastelic V, Budowle B, Drobnic K. Validation of SRY marker for forensic casework analysis. *J. Forensic Sci.* 2009 May;54(3):551-5.

Kumagai R, Sasaki Y, Tokuta T, Biwasaka H, Aoki Y. DNA analysis of family members with deletion in Yp11.2 region containing amelogenin locus. *Leg. Med.* (Tokyo). 2008 Jan;10(1):39-42.

Kumagai R, Sasaki Y, Tokuta T, Biwasaka H, Matsusue A, Aoki Y, Dewa K. Distinct breakpoints in two cases with deletion in the Yp11.2 region in Japanese population. *Hum. Genet.* 2010 Mar;127(5):537-43.

Lattanzi W, Di Giacomo MC, Lenato GM, Chimienti G, Voglino G, Resta N, Pepe G, Guanti G. A large interstitial deletion encompassing the amelogenin gene on the short arm of the Y chromosome. *Hum. Genet.* 2005 Apr;116(5):395-401.

Maciejewska A, Pawlowski R. A rare mutation in the primer binding region of the Amelogenin X homologue gene. *Forensic Sci. Int. Genet.* 2009;3:265-7.

Mannucci A, Sullivan KM, Ivanov PL, Gill P. Forensic application of a rapid and quantitative DNA sex test by amplification of the X-Y homologous gene amelogenin. *Int. J. Legal Med.* 1994;106(4):190-3.

Michael A, Brauner P. Erroneous gender identification by the amelogenin sex test. *J. Forensic Sci.* 2004;49:258-9.

Mitchell RJ, Kreskas M, Baxter E, Buffalino L, Van Oorschot RA. An investigation of sequence deletions of amelogenin (AMELY), a Y-chromosome locus commonly used for gender determination. *Ann. Hum. Biol.* 2006 Mar-Apr;33(2):227-40.

Morikawa T, Yamamoto Y, Miyaishi S. A new method for sex determination based on detection of SRY, STS and amelogenin gene regions with simultaneous amplification of their homologous sequences by a multiplex PCR. *Acta Med. Okayama.* 2011 Apr;65(2):113-22.

Mukerjee S, Mukherjee M, Ghosh T, Kalpana D, Sharma AK. Differential pattern of genetic variability at the DXYS156 locus on homologous regions of X and Y chromosomes in Indian population and its forensic implications. *Int. J. Legal Med.* 2011 Nov 25. [Epub ahead of print].

Nakahori Y, Takenaka O, Nakagome Y. A human X-Y homologous region encodes amelogenin. *Genomics.* 1991; 9:264-9.

Richard B, Delgado S, Gorry P, Sire JY. A study of polymorphism in human AMELX. *Arch. Oral Biol.* 2007 Nov;52(11):1026-31.

Roffey PE, Eckhoff CI, Kuhl JL. A rare mutation in the amelogenin gene and its potential investigative ramifications. *J. Forensic. Sci.* 2000 Sep;45(5):1016-9.

Santos FR, Pandya A, Tyler-Smith C. Reliability of DNA-based sex tests. *Nat. Genet.* 1998 Feb;18(2):103.

Shadrach B, Commane M, Hren C, Warshawsky I. A rare mutation in the primer binding region of the Amelogenin gene can interfere with gender identification. *J. Mol. Diagn.* 2004;6:401-5.

Skaletsky H, Kuroda-Kawaguchi T, Minx PJ, Cordum HS, Hillier L, Brown LG, Repping S, Pyntikova T, Ali J, Bieri T, Chinwalla A, Delehaunty A, Delehaunty K, Du H, Fewell G, Fulton L, Fulton R, Graves T, Hou SF,

Latrielle P, Leonard S, Mardis E, Maupin R, McPherson J, Miner T, Nash W, Nguyen C, Ozersky P, Pepin K, Rock S, Rohlfing T, Scott K, Schultz B, Strong C, Tin-Wollam A, Yang SP, Waterston RH, Wilson RK, Rozen S, Page DC. The male-specific region of the human Y chromosome is a mosaic of discrete sequence classes. *Nature*. 2003 Jun;423(6942):825-37.

Steinlechner M, Berger B, Niederstätter H, Parson W. Rare failures in the amelogenin sex test. *Int. J. Legal Med*. 2002 Apr;116(2):117-20.

Sullivan KM, Mannucci A, Kimpton CP, Gill P. A rapid and quantitative DNA sex test: fluorescence-based PCR analysis of X-Y homologous gene amelogenin. *Biotechniques*. 1993 Oct;15(4):636-641.

Takayama T, Takada N, Suzuki R, Nagaoka S, Watanabe Y, Kumagai R, Aoki Y, Butler JM. Determination of deleted regions from Yp11.2 of an amelogenin negative male. *Leg. Med.* (Tokyo). 2009 Apr;11 Suppl 1:S578-80.

Thangaraj K, Reddy AG, Singh L. Is the amelogenin gene reliable for gender identification in forensic casework and prenatal diagnosis? *Int. J. Legal Med.* 2002 Apr;116(2):121-3.

Turrina S, Filippini G, Voglino G, De Leo D. Two additional reports of deletion on the short arm of the Y chromosome. *Forensic Sci. Int. Genet.* 2011 Jun;5(3):242-6.

von Wurmb-Schwark N, Bosinski H, Ritz-Timme S. What do the X and Y chromosomes tell us about sex and gender in forensic case analysis? *J. Forensic Leg. Med.* 2007 Jan;14(1):27-30.

Zhu B, Sun QW, Lu YC, Sun MM, Wang LJ, Huang XH. Prenatal fetal sex diagnosis by detecting amelogenin gene in maternal plasma. *Prenat. Diagn.* 2005 Jul;25(7):577-81.

In: Sex Chromosomes: New Research
Editors: M. D'Aquino and V. Stallone
ISBN: 978-1-62417-143-7
© 2013 Nova Science Publishers, Inc.

Chapter VI

Non-invasive Prenatal Diagnosis for Fetal Sex Determination

Aggeliki Kolialexi[1,*]*, Georgia Tounta*[1]*,
Danay Mavreli*[1]*, Ariadni Mavrou*[1]
and Nikolas Papantoniou[2]

[1]Department of Medical Genetics and [2]1st Derartement of Obstetrics and Gynecology, Athens University School of Medicine, Athens, Greece

Abstract

Clinical indications for fetal sex determination include risk of X-linked disorders, a family history of conditions associated with ambiguous development of external genitalia and some fetal ultrasound findings. It is usually performed in the first trimester from fetal material obtained through CVS and is associated with an approximately 1% risk of miscarriage. Ultrasound fetal sex determination is often performed after 11 weeks of gestation.

Diagnosis of fetal sex was one of the earliest developed tests for non invasive prenatal diagnosis (NIPD) from the 7th week of gestation using cell free fetal DNA (cffDNA) circulating in maternal plasma. The majority of reported studies are based on quantitative real-time PCR (RT-

---

[*] Corresponding author: Aggeliki Kolialexi, Medical Genetics, Athens University School of Medicine, Athens Greece. Tel: 210 7467462; Fax: 210 7795553; E-mail: akolial@med.uoa.gr.

qPCR) analysis of the SRY gene, achieving sensitivities of 90–100%, with an extremely low incidence of false positive results. False negative results are usually due to failure of amplification of the SRY gene in male fetuses caused by undetectable levels of cffDNA in maternal plasma. A gender independent fetal marker is therefore necessary to verify the presence of fetal DNA sequences. Female fetuses are not detected directly, but by the absence of Y chromosome specific sequences.

Fetal sex determination by cffDNA analysis is currently performed clinically in many centers in order to avoid conventional invasive testing in pregnant women at risk for X-linked and endocrinal disorder.

Introduction

At present, prenatal fetal gender determination is performed in the 1st trimester of pregnancy using fetal genetic material obtained through chorionic villus sampling (CVS). This invasive procedure, however, has a low but definite risk of around 1% for miscarriage [1, 2].

Non invasive fetal sex determination can be carried out using ultrasonography, which is accurate after 12 weeks as the morphological appearance of the male and female external genitalia is similar before 12 weeks of gestation [3]. As CVS can be offered at 11 weeks, sex determination at 12 weeks and beyond is too late for those women who would like to have early definitive genetic diagnosis. In addition, where there is a risk of genital ambiguity, ultrasound cannot be used reliably at any week of gestation. Thus alternative sources of fetal material have been investigated to allow early and accurate non-invasive fetal gender determination.

One approach is based on the isolation of fetal nucleated cells from the maternal circulation [4]. This investigation, however, has not been successful, since it is difficult to isolate and analyse intact fetal cells and may not be pregnancy specific [5, 6].

In 1997, Lo et al. identified the presence of cell-free fetal DNA (cffDNA) in maternal plasma [7]. Following this early work, a number of papers have described the physical features of cffDNA and its use for NIPD. CffDNA is found in the plasma of all pregnant women from 4–5 weeks of pregnancy with an increasing percentage along gestation [8]. Furthermore, it rapidly disappears from maternal circulation following delivery [9]. Studies regarding the size distribution of cffDNA have confirmed that it is of average size 300 bp or smaller, in contrast to maternal cffDNA fragments, which are considerably larger [10, 11]. Data support the theory that the placenta is the major source of cffDNA molecules [12-14].

Most cfDNA in the circulation is of maternal origin. Digital polymerase chain reaction (PCR) has allowed precise quantification of cfDNA levels, showing that the fetal component contributes around 9% in early pregnancy, increasing to 20% as the pregnancy progresses [15]. The relative proportion of fetal DNA in maternal plasma is known to increase in certain pregnancy complications, including preeclampsia and fetal aneuploidies [16, 17].

The key limiting factor in the development of specific prenatal tests based on cffDNA has been the difficulty to differentiate fetal genetic material from that of the mother. As a result, the first clinical applications of NIPD have been restricted to the identification of alleles present in the fetus but not in the mother (either inherited from the father or *de novo*). These include fetal sex determination, fetal RhD status and paternally inherited single-gene disorders, or those arising *de novo*, such as achondroplasia.

In this chapter we consider the impact of cffDNA for non invasive fetal sex determination in clinical practice and discuss the diagnostic issues that may arise.

Indications for Fetal Gender Determination

X-Linked Disorders

The most common clinical indication for early fetal sex assessment is for carriers of X-linked genetic disorders, such as haemophilia and Duchenne muscular dystrophy (DMD), where male-bearing pregnancies are primarily at risk [18]. Although each disease is individually relatively rare, it has been estimated that their cumulative incidence is around 5 in 10 000 live births [19]. For women carriers of X-linked conditions, early fetal sex determination using cffDNA can indicate the uptake of invasive testing. If a male fetus is identified, the woman can have invasive prenatal testing at 11 weeks for definitive diagnosis of the condition. If a female fetus is identified, an invasive test is not needed and the associated miscarriage risk can be avoided.

Congenital Adrenal Hyperplasia

Another key clinical indication for early fetal sex determination is for pregnancies at risk of congenital adrenal hyperplasia (CAH). Congenital adrenal hyperplasia (CAH) is a group of autosomal recessive disorders of cortisol biosynthesis. The deficiency of 21-hydroxylase, which accounts for approximately 95% of CAH cases, results in overproduction of adrenal androgens and exposure to excess androgens can cause ambiguous genitalia in female fetuses [20]. Since the genitalia of a female fetus may become virilised from 6 weeks after conception, it is currently recommended that maternal dexamethasone administration should begin from 6–7 weeks of gestation, in order to reduce the genital ambiguity in affected female fetuses [21] CVS is then recommended at 11 weeks to detect the gender of the fetus and disease status and treatment can be discontinued if the results show a male or an unaffected female fetus [22]. As fetal sex determination by cffDNA analysis can be performed from about the 7th week of gestation, the duration of unnecessary dexamethasone treatment in male fetuses can be shortene [23].

Genital Ambiguity

Fetal sex determination using cffDNA can also be useful in the clarification of some fetal ultrasound findings. These include confirmation of genetic sex, if abnormal genitalia are identified and additional information for diagnosing genetic conditions where genital ambiguity or sex reversal is a feature of the condition [24].

Technical Issues

Since the placenta is the major source of cffDNA molecules, ultrasonography before blood sampling, with particular attention for the presence of a second gestational sac is recommended in order to exclude the possibility of a vanishing male twin which can cause false positive results [25].

Sample processing protocols clearly affect the quantity and quality of cffDNA obtained and accordingly fetal gender determination. Although some researchers did not find any differences in detection of fetal sequences using either plasma or serum, it has been reported that cffDNA levels are double in the plasma and the excess of maternal cfDNA is much lower as compared to serum [26].

Although concentrations of cfDNA in maternal plasma have been shown to be considerably stable, it is highly recommended that blood processing takes place as soon as possible after sampling in order to prevent lysis of maternal cell [24, 27, 28]. Therefore, it is common practice for maternal blood to be processed in less than 48h after sampling. Prompt preparation of plasma, or use of cell-stabilizing collection tubes that prevent lysis of maternal cells, is required to optimize the proportion of cffDNA [29]. Plasma is removed by centrifugation and a second centrifugation at high speed or a filtration is considered essential in order to remove all cellular material. Centrifugation, however, is usually preferred because it is simpler and has a lower cost than filtration [30].

Partners of the Special Non-Invasive Advances in Fetal and Neonatal Evaluation Network of Excellence (SAFE NoE) identified the most promising protocol for the extraction of cffDNA from maternal plasma. They demonstrated that QIAamp DSP Virus Kit (Qiagen) is the optimal candidate for a manual reference method. One likely reason for the increased amount of cffDNA obtained by the QIAamp DSP Virus Kit is that this is designed to extract mainly short fragments of genomic DNA (<300 bp) [10, 11].

NIPD for fetal gender determination is performed by targeting Y-chromosome-specific sequences in maternal plasma. The majority of reports have used detection of the Y-chromosome gene *SRY* or the DYS14 marker sequence of the *TSPY* gene. Detection of a single copy sequence such as SRY could be difficult during the first trimester of pregnancy because of the low copy number of foetal DNA molecules in the plasma. The DYS14 sequence is present in multiple copies and is therefore easier to detect in maternal plasma when a male fetus is present, having a 10-fold lower detection limit than SRY [31]. The DYS14 assay has a higher sensitivity than SRY, but sometime gives false-positive results. Homologies between DYS14 primers and probe and sequences on chromosomes other than Y, lead to non-specific amplification [31]. In low DNA template reactions, several factors can lead to less efficient or unspecific amplification of the high background of maternal DNA [31, 32].

Conventional PCR, followed by agarose gel electrophoresis to visualize the PCR product, was used in the first report of the detection of fetal Y-chromosome DNA in maternal plasma. In order to increase the sensitivity of diagnosis nested PCR was also applied [33]. This nested PCR assay involves two PCRs, the first for the amplification of a specific region of SRY and the second, using the PCR product from the first round as a template, to amplify a smaller region of the gene, within the boundaries of the primary PCR primer positions.

Currently, almost all laboratories carrying out non invasive fetal gender determination using ccfDNA extracted from maternal plasma use real-time quantitative polymerase chain reaction (qRTPCR) technology with Taqman chemistry. The main advantages of qRTPCR over conventional PCR are that it is quantitative, making it easy to distinguish fetal and maternal contributions and the amplification and analysis take place in closed tubes, reducing the risks of contamination. A correlation between Ct value and week of gestation is observed because the concentration of cffDNA increases with gestational age. The wide range of Ct values in each qRT-PCR and the poor repeatability of some replicates are partly attributed to individual sampling variation in the extracted cfDNA or differences in the efficiency and sensitivity of each qRT-PCR assay. These data highlight the importance of performing several replicates from each maternal sample.

Detection of Y Chromosome-specific Sequences in Maternal Plasma

A recent systematic review and meta-analysis identified 57 studies published since the late 1990s describing the use of cffDNA for fetal sex determination in 3524 male and 3017 female-bearing pregnancies [18]. This meta-analysis showed that the test has 94.8% sensitivity and 98.9% specificity between 7 and 12 weeks increasing to a sensitivity of 99% and specificity of 99.6% after 20 weeks.

There are two concerns regarding the NIPD of fetal gender using cffDNA. The first is the possibility for false-negative results, as female fetuses are identified through a negative result, which could also be caused by insufficient cffDNA present in the assay. The second concern is the failure rate of individual tests of 5% reported in many studies [18, 25]. It is important therefore to confirm the presence of cffDNA in maternal plasma when a negative result for Y chromosome sequences is obtained. A panel of 24 bi-insertion/deletion polymorphic markers or paternally inherited blood group antigens has been used to demonstrate the presence of cffDNA [32]. Such genetic variation–based approaches, however, are time-consuming because maternal and paternal DNA must be first typed to ensure that at least one marker is informative and therefore may facilitate analysis [34].

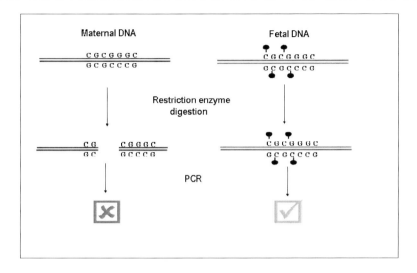

Figure 1. The promoter of RASSF1A is methylated in the placenta and unmethylated in maternal blood cells. Following restriction digestion with methylation specific enzymes, maternal DNA is digested and cannot be amplified by PCR. Fetal DNA remains undigested and can be amplified by PCR.

Alternatively, an epigenetic approach can be applied. It has been reported that DNA methylation pattern differs between the placenta and maternal blood cells. DNA methylation refers to the presence of a methyl group on the 50 carbon typically of a cytosine nucleotide that precedes a guanine nucleotide, i.e. a CpG dinucleotide. CpG methylation in the promoter regions of genes are involved in the regulation of gene expression. As tissues in the body have different gene expression profiles, the methylation status of certain genes also exhibits tissue-specific patterns.

The maspin gene promoter (*SERPINB5*) for example was methylated in maternal blood cells and hypomethylated in the placenta [14]. Placental-derived hypomethylated maspin was detectable in maternal plasma regardless the fetal sex and genetic variations and thus could serve as a universal fetal DNA marker. Detection, however, of unmethylated maspin sequences in maternal plasma requires bisulfite treatment of the sample which can lead to DNA degradation of up to 96% [14, 35]. Differential methylation status between maternal red blood cells and fetal tissues in the promoter of the *RASSF1A* gene has also been reported [36]. *RASSF1A* is hypermethylated in placenta but hypomethylated in maternal blood cells. In this case, use of a methylation-sensitive endonuclease can digest maternal hypomethylated *RASSF1A* sequences, leaving intact for amplification sequences of placental origin (figure 1). Recently a multiplex PCR-based protocol that involves *RASSF1A* amplification, in order to confirm the presence of cffDNA, was reported for fetal sex determination using cffDNA from maternal plasma [37]. This multiplex PCR was designed to allow for the simultaneous amplification of two Y chromosome specific sequences (*SRY* and *DYS14*), *RASSF1A* and *ACTB*. *ACTB* was used as an internal control system for the detection of incomplete enzyme digestion, which could potentially lead to false-positive results [36]. Stringent criteria in reporting a male bearing pregnancy were used. Following enzyme digestion, using a methylation specific restriction enzyme, this multiplex PCR assay directly demonstrates the presence of cffDNA, provides reassurance in the test result and prevents reporting of false negative results. The sensitivity and specificity of the test at 6-12 weeks of gestation was shown to be 100%. To minimize sample contamination, however, precautions should be most stringent and even the cfDNA isolation kit reagents should be aliquoted and used once by properly trained personnel.

Conclusion

NIPD can provide clinical benefits in many women by avoiding the risks of invasive testing. In Europe fetal sex determination is available as early as 7 weeks of gestation. The test must be ordered through a physician and has sensitivity and specificity of 97% based on large-scale validation studies. Parents should be advised of the small risk of discordant results and of the possibility that repeat testing may be required to resolve inconclusive results.

There is no additional cost to health services since higher testing costs associated with NIPD are compensated by the fact that fewer women require invasive testing [38]. An ultrasound scan should be used to confirm the gestation and check for twin pregnancies before blood sampling and should also be offered following NIPD to confirm fetal gender reported using cffDNA.

Acknowledgment

The first two authors contributed equally to the study and should be both considered as first author. Funding from the European Commission for the Special Non-Invasive Advances in Fetal and Neonatal Evaluation (SAFE)

Network of Excellence (LSHB-CT-2004- 503243) for which this study was funded is gratefully acknowledged.

References

[1] Mujezinovic, F; Alfirevic, Z. Procedure-related complications of amniocentesis and chorionic villous sampling: a systematic review. *Obstet Gynecol*, 2007 110(3), 687-94.
[2] Wald, N and Leck, I. *Antenatal and Neonatal Screening*. 2nd ed. 2000, Oxford University Press: Oxford:. 1-57.
[3] Efrat, Z; Perri, T; Ramati, E; Tugendreich, D; Meizner, I. Fetal gender assignment by first-trimester ultrasound. *Ultrasound Obstet Gynecol*, 2006 27(6), 619-21.
[4] Bianchi, D. W; Flint, A. F; Pizzimenti, M. F; Knoll, J. H; Latt, S. A. Isolation of fetal DNA from nucleated erythrocytes in maternal blood. *Proc Natl Acad Sci U S A*, 1990 87(9), 3279-83.
[5] Bianchi, D. W; Wataganara, T; Lapaire, O; Tjoa, M. L; Maron, J. L; Larrabee, P. B; Johnson, K. L. Fetal nucleic acids in maternal body fluids: an update. *Ann N Y Acad Sci*, 2006 1075, 63-73.
[6] Bianchi, D. W. Prenatal diagnosis: we are the future. *Prenat Diagn*, 2007 27(10), 891-2.
[7] Lo, Y. M; Corbetta, N; Chamberlain, P. F; Rai, V; Sargent, I. L; Redman, C. W; Wainscoat, J. S. Presence of fetal DNA in maternal plasma and serum. *Lancet*, 1997 350(9076), 485-7.
[8] Rijnders, R. J; van der Luijt, R. B; Peters, E. D; Goeree, J. K; van der Schoot, C. E; Ploos van Amstel, J. K; Christiaens, G. C. Earliest gestational age for fetal sexing in cell-free maternal plasma. *Prenat Diagn*, 2003 23(13), 1042-4.
[9] Lo, Y. M; Zhang, J; Leung, T. N; Lau, T. K; Chang, A. M; Hjelm, N. M. Rapid clearance of fetal DNA from maternal plasma. *Am J Hum Genet*, 1999 64(1), 218-24.
[10] Chan, K. C; Zhang, J; Hui, A. B; Wong, N; Lau, T. K; Leung, T. N; Lo, K. W; Huang, D. W; Lo, Y. M. Size distributions of maternal and fetal DNA in maternal plasma. *Clin Chem*, 2004 50(1), 88-92.
[11] Li, Y; Zimmermann, B; Rusterholz, C; Kang, A; Holzgreve, W; Hahn, S. Size separation of circulatory DNA in maternal plasma permits ready detection of fetal DNA polymorphisms. *Clin Chem*, 2004 50(6), 1002-11.

[12] Lui, Y. Y; Woo, K. S; Wang, A. Y; Yeung, C. K; Li, P. K; Chau, E; Ruygrok, P; Lo, Y. M. Origin of plasma cell-free DNA after solid organ transplantation. *Clin Chem*, 2003 49(3), 495-6.
[13] Ng, E. K; Tsui, N. B; Lau, T. K; Leung, T. N; Chiu, R. W; Panesar, N. S; Lit, L. C; Chan, K. W; Lo, Y. M. mRNA of placental origin is readily detectable in maternal plasma. *Proc Natl Acad Sci U S A*, 2003 100(8), 4748-53.
[14] Chim, S. S; Tong, Y. K; Chiu, R. W; Lau, T. K; Leung, T. N; Chan, L. Y; Oudejans, C. B; Ding, C; Lo, Y. M. Detection of the placental epigenetic signature of the maspin gene in maternal plasma. *Proc Natl Acad Sci U S A*, 2005 102(41), 14753-8.
[15] Lun, F. M; Chiu, R. W; Allen Chan, K. C; Yeung Leung, T; Kin Lau, T; Dennis Lo, Y. M. Microfluidics digital PCR reveals a higher than expected fraction of fetal DNA in maternal plasma. *Clin Chem*, 2008 54(10), 1664-72.
[16] Hahn, S; Chitty, L. S. Noninvasive prenatal diagnosis: current practice and future perspectives. *Curr Opin Obstet Gynecol*, 2008 20(2), 146-51.
[17] Lo, Y. M. Fetal nucleic acids in maternal plasma. *Ann N Y Acad Sci*, 2008 1137, 140-3.
[18] Devaney, S. A; Palomaki, G. E; Scott, J. A; Bianchi, D. W. Noninvasive fetal sex determination using cell-free fetal DNA: a systematic review and meta-analysis. *JAMA*, 2011 306(6), 627-36.
[19] Baird, P. A; Anderson, T. W; Newcombe, H. B; Lowry, R. B. Genetic disorders in children and young adults: a population study. *Am J Hum Genet*, 1988 42(5), 677-93.
[20] Merke, D. P; Bornstein, SR. Congenital adrenal hyperplasia. *Lancet*, 2005 365(9477), 2125-36.
[21] Speiser, P. W; Azziz, R; Baskin, L. S; Ghizzoni, L; Hensle, T. W; Merke, D. P; Meyer-Bahlburg, H. F; Miller, W. L; Montori, V. M; Oberfield, S. E; Ritzen, M; White, P. C. Congenital adrenal hyperplasia due to steroid 21-hydroxylase deficiency: an Endocrine Society clinical practice guideline. *J Clin Endocrinol Metab*, 2010 95(9), 4133-60.
[22] Nimkarn, S; New, M. I. Prenatal diagnosis and treatment of congenital adrenal hyperplasia due to 21-hydroxylase deficiency. *Mol Cell Endocrinol*, 2009 300(1-2), 192-6.
[23] Bartha, J. L; Finning, K; Soothill, P. W. Fetal sex determination from maternal blood at 6 weeks of gestation when at risk for 21-hydroxylase deficiency. *Obstet Gynecol*, 2003 101(5 Pt 2), 1135-6.

[24] Finning, K. M; Chitty, L. S. Non-invasive fetal sex determination: impact on clinical practice. *Semin Fetal Neonatal Med*, 2008 13(2), 69-75.

[25] Hill, M; Finning, K; Martin, P; Hogg, J; Meaney, C; Norbury, G; Daniels, G; Chitty, L. S. Non-invasive prenatal determination of fetal sex: translating research into clinical practice. *Clin Genet*, 2011 80(1), 68-75.

[26] Houfflin-Debarge, V; O'Donnell, H; Overton, T; Bennett, P. R; Fisk, N. M. High sensitivity of fetal DNA in plasma compared to serum and nucleated cells using unnested PCR in maternal blood. *Fetal Diagn Ther*, 2000 15(2), 102-7.

[27] Angert, R. M; LeShane, E. S; Lo, Y. M; Chan, L. Y; Delli-Bovi, L. C; Bianchi, D. W. Fetal cell-free plasma DNA concentrations in maternal blood are stable 24 hours after collection: analysis of first- and third-trimester samples. *Clin Chem*, 2003 49(1), 195-8.

[28] Minon, J. M; Gerard, C; Senterre, J. M; Schaaps, J. P; Foidart, J. M. Routine fetal RHD genotyping with maternal plasma: a four-year experience in Belgium. *Transfusion*, 2008 48(2), 373-81.

[29] Barrett, A. N; Zimmermann, B. G; Wang, D; Holloway, A; Chitty, LS. Implementing prenatal diagnosis based on cell-free fetal DNA: accurate identification of factors affecting fetal DNA yield. *PLoS One*, 2011 6(10), e25202.

[30] Chiu, R. W; Poon, L. L; Lau, T. K; Leung, T. N; Wong, E. M; Lo, Y. M. Effects of blood-processing protocols on fetal and total DNA quantification in maternal plasma. *Clin Chem*, 2001 47(9), 1607-13.

[31] Zimmermann, B; El-Sheikhah, A; Nicolaides, K; Holzgreve, W; Hahn, S. Optimized real-time quantitative PCR measurement of male fetal DNA in maternal plasma. *Clin Chem*, 2005 51(9), 1598-604.

[32] Scheffer, P. G; van der Schoot, C. E; Page-Christiaens, G. C; Bossers, B; van Erp, F; de Haas, M. Reliability of fetal sex determination using maternal plasma. *Obstet Gynecol*, 2010 115(1), 117-26.

[33] Zhong, X. Y; Holzgreve, W; Hahn, S. Detection of fetal Rhesus D and sex using fetal DNA from maternal plasma by multiplex polymerase chain reaction. *BJOG*, 2000 107(6), 766-9.

[34] Page-Christiaens, G. C; Bossers, B; Ce, V. D. S;, Deh M. Use of bi-allelic insertion/deletion polymorphisms as a positive control for fetal genotyping in maternal blood: first clinical experience. *Ann N Y Acad Sci*, 2006 1075, 123-9.

[35] Grunau, C; Clark, S. J; Rosenthal, A. Bisulfite genomic sequencing: systematic investigation of critical experimental parameters. *Nucleic Acids Res*, 2001 29(13), E65-5.
[36] Chan, K. C; Ding, C; Gerovassili, A; Yeung, S. W; Chiu, R. W; Leung, T. N; Lau, T. K; Chim, S, S; Chung, G. T; Nicolaides, K. H; Lo, Y. M. Hypermethylated RASSF1A in maternal plasma: A universal fetal DNA marker that improves the reliability of noninvasive prenatal diagnosis. *Clin Chem*, 2006 52(12), 2211-8.
[37] Kolialexi, A; Tounta, G; Apostolou, P; Vrettou, C; Papantoniou, N; Kanavakis, E; Antsaklis, A; Mavrou, A. Early non-invasive detection of fetal Y chromosome sequences in maternal plasma using multiplex PCR. *Eur J Obstet Gynecol Reprod Biol*, 2012 161(1), 34-7.
[38] Hill, M; Taffinder, S; Chitty, L. S; Morris, S. Incremental cost of non-invasive prenatal diagnosis versus invasive prenatal diagnosis of fetal sex in England. *Prenat Diagn*, 2011 31(3), 267-73.

In: Sex Chromosomes: New Research
Editors: M. D'Aquino and V. Stallone

ISBN: 978-1-62417-143-7
© 2013 Nova Science Publishers, Inc.

Chapter VII

Application of X Chromosomal STR Polymorphisms to Individual Identification

Jian Tie[*] *and Seisaku Uchigasaki*
Division of Legal Medicine, Department of Social Medicine,
Nihon University School of Medicine
Itabashi-ku, Tokyo Japan

Abstract

The human DNA markers most commonly utilized in individual identification are autosomal short tandem repeat (STR), followed by Y-chromosome STRs and mitochondrial DNA. X-chromosomal short tandem repeat (X-STR) loci may efficiently complement autosomal markers in paternity testing, especially in deficient paternity cases with female offspring, and in kinship analysis involving large and incomplete pedigrees. X-STR loci are located on the non-recombining region of the X chromosome and are inherited as a block of linked haplotypes. Due to its unique inheritance pattern, the X chromosome is a potential candidate for forensic and human identity testing applications. Currently, more than 40 X-STRs have been established as forensic markers, and a large number of population data have been published. X-STR haplotyping can

---

[*] Phone: +81-3-3972-8111, Fax: +81-3-3958-7776, Email: tetsu.ken@nihon-u.ac.jp.

be of particular help in kinship testing in deficient paternity cases where a DNA sample from one of the parents is not available for testing. The ideal technique for X-STR typing is multiplex PCR, because as the number of polymorphic loci examined increases, the probability of identical alleles being present in two different individuals decreases. Multiplex systems have been developed in order to apply X-STRs efficiently for paternity testing. In view of the wide application of these markers, several X-STRs multiplex PCR systems have been validated for individual identification, which include four to thirty markers. Multiplex with greater number of markers are being developed to obtain a high degree of discrimination. Samples from a mass disaster site or from a crime scene exposed to environment are often not only highly degraded but also in very scarce quantities, making it difficult for scientists to perform multiple PCR analyses. Analysis of degraded DNA samples using mini X-STR multiplex systems will offer high efficacy for personal identification.

Introduction

In the early 1990s, short tandem repeats (STR) markers were first reported as effective tools for human identity testing [1, 2]. Forensic scientists began to aggressively search for new loci and study population variations. Performance studies and protocol evaluations were performed; population databases were established; and forensic validation was conducted on the various STR systems investigated. The X-chromosomal (ChrX) STR (X-STR) has recently been recognized to be useful tools in forensic medicine and anthropological studies for human identification as well as kinship and paternity testing, mainly in deficient paternity cases when the disputed child is a female [3, 4]. The distinctive properties of inheritance of the ChrX are responsible for its importance in population genetic studies. Features of X-chromosomal inheritance that are relevant to forensic casework will be discussed on the basis of empirical data.

In the cells of healthy human females, the ChrX are present as a homologous pair and resemble autosomes in this respect [2]. For a given pair of parents, the presence of gonosomal irregularities can usually be excluded since these would be associated with infertility.

Unexpected and undetected aberrant gonosomal karyotypes may however occur in the offspring, thereby affecting the accuracy of kinship testing using ChrX markers.

X-STR Markers in Forensic Science

The first significant achievement in X-chromosomal markers was made when the Xga blood group was detected by the team of Race and Sanger. A review on this topic has been published by Tippett and Ellis [5]. The first two ChrX microsatellites that played a significant role were HPRTB [2, 6] and ARA [2, 7]. One of the challenges in kinship testing is to establish techniques that can bridge large pedigree gaps. From observations in clinical genetics, we know that persons who share a very rare genetic feature can be combined into a common pedigree. The approach of substituting single STRs by haplotypes consisting of clustered STR may also provide highly indicative tools, and can be systematically applied to forensic studies.

Paternity Testing

Autosomal STR is usually the first choice for paternity cases involving the common trio constellation of mother, offspring and alleged father. However, when father/daughter relationship is to be tested, it may be worthwhile to include X-STR. In other special cases such as a man who married two women each of whom had a daughter. After the man died, to test if the two daughters have the same father, mitochondrial DNA marker cannot be used for identification because they come from different mothers. In this case, X-STR is useful for paternity testing. For testing mother-daughter relationship, X-STR are equivalent to autosomal STR and do not confer any specific advantage. Testing mother-son kinship, however, is more efficiently performed using X-STR. This is especially the case when there are difficulties in analyzing template materials, such as DNA from exhumed skeletons or historic or prehistoric samples.

Criminal Casework

As the forensic techniques advance, so do the techniques of the perpetrators of crimes. Moreover, industrialization of our world further confounds the evidence found at a crime scene or the samples left at a mass disaster site. Hence, there is a constant pressure to develop novel and precise methods to arrest the guilty but to exonerate the innocent, or to accurately identify a missing relative. From fingerprinting to DNA profiling, many techniques were standardized and discarded until we arrived at databasing of core STR loci. Since then, millions of profiles have been generated, and it is very likely that STR will be the workhorse for the foreseeable future [8].

Pregnancies resulting from criminal sexual assault or incest may be terminated by suction abortion. A several-week-old aborted product of conception consists of small amounts of non-identifiable fetal organs as well as maternal blood and other tissues. In such cases, microscopic dissection of chorionic villi is usually not successful, and samples most often contain a mixture of fetal and maternal DNA. Efficient paternity testing of such material is still possible for male fetuses, using Y chromosomal STR. Paternity testing of female fetuses, in contrast, relies only on autosomal and X-STR, the latter representing a more efficient means of paternity exclusion under all circumstances. In incest cases in which a father is rightfully charged with abusing his daughter, X-STR testing of an abortus provides only very limited information toward a positive proof of paternity. This is because all fetal alleles would necessarily coincide with alleles of the daughter.

In other words, X-STRs are less powerful in analyzing forensic samples than autosomal STRs, because X-STR analysis in males utilizes only one allele per STR. However, in a mixed female/male stain, the chance of all male alleles being included in the female component is higher for X-STR than for autosomal STR.

Detection of X-STR and Advances

While early works with STR involved detection on silver-stained polyacrylamide gels [9], the human identity testing community gradually embraced fluorescence detection methods involving gel electrophoresis [2, 10, 11] followed by capillary electrophoresis with instruments such as the ABI 310 and other genetic analyzers [12]. For autosomal STR multiplex analysis, several commercial kits detecting over 13 loci and the amelogenin sex-typing system in one tube using multiplex PCR amplification have become available. A multiplex PCR system that co-amplifies multiple X-STR markers has become an attractive tool for genetic and forensic investigations. Recently multiplex PCR systems for analyzing X-STR have been used to study several populations [13, 14]. Mentype Argus (Biotype, AG, Dresden, Germany) has developed a multiplex kit for analyzing eight X-STR loci and amelogenin. In addition, a new twelve X-STR multiplex amplification kit (Investigator Argus X-12, QIAGEN) has also become available (Table 1).

Table 1. X-STR genotyping using commercial kits

Locus	Mentype Argus	Investigator Argus X-12	Linkage group
DXS10135	+	+	1
DXS8378	+	+	1
DXS7132	+	+	2
DXS10074	+	+	2
HPRTB	+	+	3
DXS10101	+	+	3
DXS10134	+	+	4
DXS7423	+	+	4
DXS10079		+	2
DXS10103		+	3
DXS10146		+	4
DXS10148		+	1
Amelogenin	+	+	

+: The locus was included in the kit.

The four new X-STR loci included in the Investigator Argus X-12 the kit have shown higher genetic polymorphisms in several populations [15, 16].

Haplotype Analysis of X-STR

If markers are linked, they do not segregate independently. For practical purposes, the X-STR has been divided into several linkage groups that yield independent genotypes. For example, Investigator Argus X-12 kit is a valuable tool for X-STR haplotyping. In this kit, 12 X-STR loci are divided to four linkage groups (Figure 1). Generally, alleles of linked loci form haplotypes that recombine during meiosis at a frequency corresponding to the inter-marker genetic distance. For ChrX markers, this phenomenon is limited to female meiosis. We have investigated twelve X-STR haplotypes in Japanese and Chinese males, and found different linked characteristics in the haplotype profiles of the two populations (Table 2). In kinship testing, haplotypes of closely linked STR must therefore be analyzed as a group, rather than as individual alleles. The use of X-STR requires precise knowledge of not only the allele and haplotype frequencies, but also the genetic linkage and linkage disequilibrium (LD) status among markers [17].

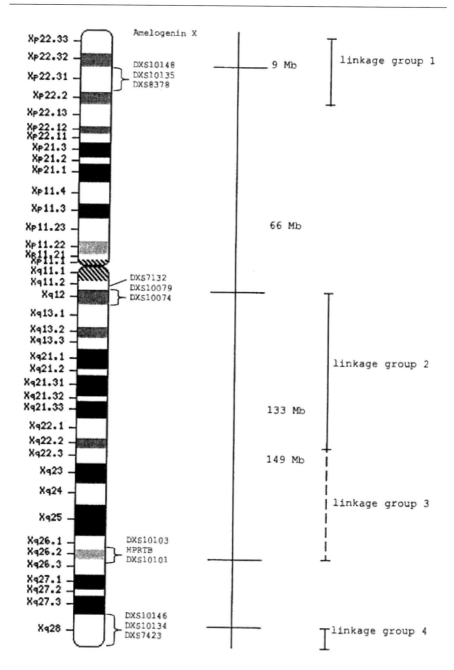

Figure 1. Location and combination of linked X-STR loci on X chromosome.

Table 2. Comparison of specific haplotypes in several populations

Linkage group	Haplotype frequencies (%)					
	Japanese	Chinese	Germany [32]	Hungary [33]	Sweden [34]	Morocco [35]
Group 1						
19-19-10	1.37	0	0	0	0	0
25.1-19-10	1.60	0	0.19	0	0.15	0
25.1-25-10	0	1.52	0.87	1.37	0.92	
27.1-20-10	0	1.52	0.19	0.46	0.46	0
Group 2					*	
14-17-18	0	2.28	0.48	0.46		0
Group 3					*	
16-12-33	1.83	0	0	0		0
16-14-30	0	1.90	0.19	0		0
19-11-32	0	2.66	0	0		0
19-12-33	1.83	0	0	0		0
19-14-32	0	1.52	0.19	0		0
Group 4					*	
26-36-14	1.37	0	0.48	0.46		0
29-36-16	1.37	0	0.58	0		0

*Data not available.

For X-STR, differences in allele distribution are marginal if closely related populations are compared. However, if investigation is conducted in a worldwide context, different populations may show significant differences in their allele frequency.

Linkage disequilibrium (LD), or the non-random association of allele, is not completely understood in the human genome. However, studies of LD between microsatellites have provided new insights into the origin and history of human populations.

X-Chromosomal MiniSTR

In forensic casework, we often encounter samples that are not in the best of conditions, and consist of DNA that is highly fragmented or damaged. Typical degraded samples include bones, teeth, burnt tissues, and tissues exposed to heat and humidity. DNA molecules that are exposed to water and/or heat will over time begin to break down into smaller pieces. Nucleases from within the cell attack the DNA as soon as the cell dies, leading to degradation [18]. This degradation can also occur due to microbial, biochemical or oxidative processes. In favorable environment, microbes feed on the hydrocarbons of DNA rendering it highly fragmented. Bacteria are the main degrading agents on land while fungi are responsible for oceanic degradation [19, 20]. Traditional STR typing can cope with slightly degraded samples, but as the fragmentation increases, even traditional STR markers may yield a negative result [21-23]. Conventional STR have a size range of 100-400 bp, most of which consists of flanking sequences on both sides of the repeat region. One method to detect X-STR more effectively in degraded samples is to design primers targeting as close as possible only the STR region leaving out the extra sequences [24]. The first "pure" miniX-STR multiplex systems were reported by Asamura et al. [22], who devised two mini-multiplex PCR systems consisting of DXS7423, DXS6789, DXS101, GATA31E08, DXS8378, DXS7133, DXS7424, and GATA165B12 at X-linked STR loci. They concluded that analysis by these miniX-STR multiplex systems offers high effectiveness for personal identification from degraded DNA samples [25].

Mutation Rates of X-STR

Allelic mutations of the autosomal STRs have been reported at several loci, and precise mutation rate estimates are a prerequisite of reliable kinship testing using genetic markers. However, since X-STR not yet widely used in forensic practice, systematic investigations of X-STR mutation rates are lacking. So far, X-STR mutations have been reported only from Germany populations, based on analyses of 17 X-STR loci [26].

Discussion

X-chromosomal STR offers a new potential tool that provides distinct useful supplementary information in some forensic casework to generate full genetic profiles. Although their hereditary uniqueness render them particularly suitable for kinship testing, X-STR have so far been employed only rarely in forensic practice. This notwithstanding, since gonosomal markers are especially efficient for solving deficient paternity cases, an increasing demand of X-STR analysis can be expected. The X-STR multiplex systems are valuable for the analyses of samples where allele dropout and reduced sensitivity of larger STR alleles occur. They are also useful for improving the power of exclusion in cases where there are insufficient family references for association in mass disasters. In complex paternity cases, these loci may provide additional discrimination in parentage analysis. It should be kept in mind that the purpose of these X-STRs are not to replace but to supplement the current battery of autosomal core loci, when samples are degraded or when there is insufficient reference materials available for identification profiles.

Due to its unique inheritance pattern, the ChrX is a potential candidate for forensic and human identity testing applications. Normal males possess one ChrX and one ChrY, whereas females possess two ChrX [25]. Currently, more than 40 X-STR have been established as forensic markers [27-30]. The majority of X-STRs can be used routinely and there are no limitations in term of their usage except HumARA, one of the established STR markers. X-STR haplotyping can be of particular help in kinship testing in deficient paternity cases where a DNA sample from one of the parents is not available for testing.

Usually ChrX markers are less powerful in stain analyses than autosomal markers and are not suitable for use in testing male traces when there is female contamination. However, ChrX markers are more powerful than autosomal markers in the identification of female traces in the presence of male contamination. The ideal technique for forensic DNA typing is multiplex PCR, because as the number of polymorphic loci examined increases, the probability of identical alleles being present in two different individuals decreases [31]. Multiplex systems have been developed in order to apply the X-STR efficiently for paternity testing.

References

[1] Edwards A, Civitello A, Hammond HA, Caskey CT. DNA typing and genetic mapping with trimeric and tetrameric tandem repeats. *Am. J. Hum. Genet.* 1991; 49: 746-756.

[2] Edwards A, Hammond HA, Caskey CT, Chakraborty R. Genetic variation at five trimeric and tetrameric tandem repeat loci in four human population groups. *Genomics* 1992; 12: 241-253.

[3] Pinto N, Silva PV, Amorim A. A general method to assess the utility of the X-chromosomal markers in kinship testing. *Forensic Sci. Int. Genet.* 2012; 6(2): 198-207.

[4] Brenner CH. Counterexample to a kinship conjecture of Krawczak. *Forensic Sci. Int. Genet.* 2008; 2(1):75.
[5] Tippett P, Ellis NA. The Xg blood group system: a review, *Transfus Med. Rev.* 1998; 12 (4): 233-257.
[6] Hearne CM, Todd JA. Tetranucleotide repeat polymorphism at the HPRT locus. *Nucleic Acids Res.* 1991; 19 (19): 5450.
[7] Desmarais D, Zhang Y, Chakraborty R, Perreault C, Busque L. Development of a highly polymorphic STR marker for identity testing puposes at the human androgen receptor gene (HUMARA), *J. Forensic. Sci.* 1998; 43 (5): 1046-1049.
[8] Gill P, Werrett DJ, Budowle B, Guerrieri R. An assessment of whether SNPs will replace STRs in national DNA databases--joint considerations of the DNA working group of the European Network of Forensic Science Institutes (ENFSI) and the Scientific Working Group on DNA Analysis Methods (SWGDAM). *Sci. Justice* 2004; 44(1): 51-53.
[9] Lins AM, Sprecher CJ, Puers C, Schumm JW. Multiplex sets for the amplification of polymorphic short tandem repeat loci-silver stain and fluorescence detection. *Bio. Techniques* 1996; 20: 882-889.
[10] Kimpton CP, Gill P, Walton A, Urquhart A, Millican ES, Adams M. Automated DNA profiling employing multiplex amplification of short tandem repeat loci. *PCR Meth Appl.* 1993; 3: 13-22.
[11] Fregeau CJ, Fourney RM. DNA typing with fluorescently tagged short tandem repeats: a sensitive and accurate approach to human identification. *Bio. Techniques* 1993; 15: 100-119.
[12] Butler JM, Buel E, Crivellente F, McCord BR. Forensic DNA typing by capillary electrophoresis using the ABI Prism 310 and 3100 genetic analyzers for STR analysis. *Electrophoresis* 2004; 25: 1397-1412.
[13] Ribeiro-Rodrigues EM, Palha Tde J, Bittencourt EA, Ribeiro-Dos-Santos A, Santos S. Extensive survey of 12 X-STRs reveals genetic heterogeneity among Brazilian populations. *Int. J. Legal Med* 2011; 125: 445-452.
[14] Tie J, Uchigasaki S, Oshida S. Genetic polymorphisms of eight X-Chromosomal STR loci in the population of Japanese. *Forensic Sci. Int. Genetics* 2010; 4: e105-108.
[15] Zhang S, Zhao S, Zhu R, Li C. Genetic polymorphisms of 12 X-STR for forensic purposes in Shanghai Han population from China. *Mol. Biol. Rep.* 2012; 39(5): 5705-5707.

[16] Horváth G, Zalán A, Kis Z, Pamjav H. A genetic study of 12 X-STR loci in the Hungarian population. *Forensic Sci. Int. Genet.* 2012; 6(1): e46-47.
[17] Freitas NS, Resque RL, Ribeiro-Rodrigues EM, Guerreiro JF, Santos NP, Ribeiro-dos-Santos A X-linked insertion/deletion polymorphisms: forensic applications of a 33-markers panel. *Int. J. Legal Med.* 2010; 124: 589-593.
[18] Vaughan AT, Betti CJ, Villalobos MJ. Surviving apoptosis. *Apoptosis.* 2002; 7(2): 173-177.
[19] Butler JM. Genetics and genomics of core short tandem repeat loci used in human identity testing. *J. Forensic Sci.* 2006; 51(2): 253-265.
[20] Leahy JG, Colwell RR. Microbial degradation of hydrocarbons in the environment. *Microbiol. Rev.* 1990; 54(3): 305-315.
[21] Grubwieser P, Muhlmann R, Berger B, Niederstatter H, Pavlic M, Parson W. A new "miniSTR-multiplex" displaying reduced amplicon lengths for the analysis of degraded DNA. *Int. J. Legal Med.* 2006; 120(2): 115-120.
[22] Holland MM, Cave CA, Holland CA, Bille TW. Development of a quality, high throughput DNA analysis procedure for skeletal samples to assist with the identification of victims from the World Trade Center attacks. *Croat Med. J.* 2003; 44(3): 264-272.
[23] Parsons TJ, Huel R, Davoren J, Katzmarzyk C, Milos A, Selmanovic A. Application of novel "mini-amplicon" STR multiplexes to high volume casework on degraded skeletal remains. *Forensic Sci. Int. Genet.* 2007; 1(2): 175-179.
[24] Butler JM, Shen Y. McCord BR. The development of reduced size STR amplicons as tools for analysis of degraded DNA. *J. Forensic Sci.* 2003; 48(5): 1054-1064.
[25] Asamura H, Sakai H, Kobayashi K, Ota M, Fukushima H. MiniX-STR multiplex system population study in Japan and application to degraded DNA analysis. *Int. J. Legal Med.* 2006; 120(3): 174-181.
[26] Fracasso T, Schürenkamp M, Brinkmann B, Hohoff C. An X-STR meiosis study in Kurds and Germans: allele frequencies and mutation rates. *Int. J. Legal Med.* 2008; 122(4): 353-356.
[27] Jędrzejczyk M, Jacewicz R, Kozdraj A, Szram S, Berent J. Application of X-STR Loci in Forensic Genetics. *Prob. Forensic Sci.* 2010; 82: 141-150.

[28] Machado FB, Medina-Acosta E. Genetic map of human X-linked microsatellites used in forensic practice. *Forensic Sci. Int. Genet.* 2009; 3(3): 202-204.
[29] Szibor R. X-chromosomal markers: past, present and future. *Forensic Sci. Int. Genet.* 2007; 1(2): 93-99.
[30] Szibor R, Hering S, Edelmann J. The HumARA genotype is linked to spinal and bulbar muscular dystrophy and some further disease risks and should no longer be used as a DNA marker for forensic purposes. *Int. J. Legal Med.* 2005; 119(3): 179-180.
[31] Edwards MC, Gibbs RA. Multiplex PCR: advantages, development, and applications. *PCR Methods Appl.* 1994; 3(4): S65-75.
[32] Edelmann J, Lutz-Bonengel S, Naue J, Hering S. X-chromosomal haplotype frequencies of four linkage groups using the Investigator Argus X-12 Kit. *Forensic Sci. Int. Genet.* 2012; 6: e24-34.
[33] Horváth G, Zalán A, Kis Z, Pamjav H. A genetic study of 12 X-STR loci in the Hungarian population. *Forensic Sci. Int. Genet.* 2012; 6: e46-47.
[34] Tillmar AO. Population genetic analysis of 12 X-STRs in Swedish population. *Forensic Sci. Int. Genet.* 2012; 6: e80-81.
[35] Bentayebi K, Picornell A, Bouabdeallah M, Castro JA, Aboukhalid R, Squalli D Genetic diversity of 12 X-chromosomal short tandem repeats in the Moroccan population. *Forensic Sci. Int. Genet.* 2012; 6: e48-49.

Index

A

access, 112
accounting, 7
acetylation, 31
achondroplasia, 141
acid, 91, 112
AD, 123, 124
adenine, 133
adrenal hyperplasia, 128, 142, 148
advancement, 31
aetiology, 77, 101
Afghanistan, 96
age, 34, 35, 57, 67, 77, 82, 122, 127
Aldrich syndrome, 128
allele, x, 23, 25, 34, 46, 51, 126, 154, 155, 157, 159, 161
alternative hypothesis, 27
alters, 86
AME, xi, 126, 132
amenorrhea, 115
amino, 91, 96, 112
amino acid, 91, 96
amniocentesis, 147
amniotic fluid, 131
anchoring, 38
androgen(s), ix, x, 98, 110, 113, 114, 115, 118, 119, 142, 160
aneuploid, 82, 122
aneuploidy, 74, 77, 79, 82

annealing, 134
annotation, 41
antigen, 8
antisense, 25, 47, 49
apoptosis, 82, 119, 161
aquarium, 99
Armenia, 96
arrest, 82, 153
assault, 127, 154
assessment, 18, 128, 141, 160
ataxia, 122
ATP, 72
autosomal recessive, 142
avian, 10, 39, 43

B

backcross, 59, 63, 64
bacteriophage, 105
Baluchistan, 96
Barr body, 22, 33
base, 127
base pair, 127
basement membrane, 117
behaviors, 67
Belgium, 149
benign, 111
bias, 9
biopsy, 120, 123
biosynthesis, 142

birds, 2, 17, 24, 44, 46
births, 141
blood, 128, 142, 143, 144, 145, 146, 147, 148, 149, 153, 154, 160
blood group, 144, 153, 160
body fluid, 147
bone(s), 61, 127, 128, 157
bone marrow, 127, 128
bone marrow transplant, 127, 128
brain, 9, 15, 16, 30, 38, 60, 97
Brazil, 109
breeding, 56, 82, 84, 98, 100
brothers, 117, 131

C

Ca^{2+}, 70
Cairo, 53
calcification(s), 117
cancer, 8, 116, 117, 118, 121, 122
capillary, 154, 160
carbon, 145
carcinoma, 115, 116, 118
cardiac muscle, 23
cartilage, 61
category d, 114
cattle, 7, 33, 34, 37
Caucasus, 96
cDNA, 11, 71
cell cycle, 30
cell differentiation, x, 47, 110, 120
cell division, 21
cell line(s), 22, 34, 45, 115, 128
cell surface, 122
centric fusion, 94
centromere, 7, 94, 96, 121
cervix, 113
challenges, 153
chiasma, 12
chicken, 6, 9, 11, 17, 18, 23, 25, 27, 36, 39, 44
children, x, 83, 125, 127, 148
chimpanzee, ix, 13, 87, 92, 102, 110
China, 96, 160
choriocarcinoma, 116, 118

chorionic villi, 154
chorionic villus sampling, 140
circulation, 140, 141
CIS, 115, 120
classes, 42, 131, 138
classification, 114, 119
cleavage, 41, 55, 74, 105
clinical application, 128, 141
cloning, 112
clusters, 12
coding, 8, 25, 27, 29, 36, 48, 49
cognitive function, 78
color, 56, 83
commercial, 132, 154, 155
communication, 72, 77
community, 154
compaction, 22, 30
comparative analysis, 35, 43
compensation, viii, 2, 14, 15, 17, 18, 19, 20, 24, 35, 42, 43, 44, 53, 83, 84
competition, 93
compilation, vii
complement, xi, 16, 127, 151
complexity, 12, 33, 35, 41
complications, 141, 147
composition, 93, 99, 113, 126
conception, 142, 154
condensation, 22, 45
conflict, 43
congenital adrenal hyperplasia, 128, 142, 148
consensus, 114
conservation, ix, 8, 21, 27, 32, 37, 48, 87, 103
contamination, 144, 146, 159
controversial, vii, 2, 16
coordination, 23
correlation(s), 82, 118, 144
cortisol, 142
cost, 143, 146, 150
crimes, 153
crossing over, 88
cryptorchidism, 116, 117, 120
CT, 147, 159
culture, 24, 68

Index

cytometry, 10
cytoplasm, 70, 72, 73, 83
cytosine, 145

D

data analysis, 15
database, 129
decay, 17, 19, 92
defects, viii, 54, 56, 62, 70, 72, 73, 75
deficiency, 44, 77, 99, 142, 148
deficit, 60
degenerate, 111
degradation, 5, 12, 13, 19, 32, 41, 145, 158, 161
demographic data, 127
Denmark, 83
derivatives, 117
detectable, 145, 148
detection, ix, x, 23, 65, 110, 115, 123, 125, 127, 132, 133, 134, 135, 137, 142, 143, 146, 147, 150, 154, 160
deviation, 17
digestion, 145, 146
diploid, 14, 20, 25, 94
diplotene, 55
disaster, xii, 152, 153
discordance, 113
discrimination, xii, 127, 152, 159
diseases, x, 125, 127, 129
disequilibrium, 155, 157
disorder, xi, 55, 116, 122, 140
displacement, 29
distribution, 38, 73, 95, 96, 104, 131, 133, 140, 157
divergence, 4, 6, 7, 11, 19, 30, 32, 92, 93, 94, 96
diversity, 47, 52, 106, 162
DNase, 50
dosage, vii, viii, 1, 13, 14, 15, 17, 18, 19, 20, 22, 24, 31, 32, 34, 35, 42, 43, 44, 45, 46, 47, 50, 51, 53, 56, 58, 60, 71, 77, 80, 100

dosage compensation, vii, 1, 14, 15, 17, 18, 19, 20, 22, 24, 25, 31, 35, 42, 43, 44, 45, 46, 47, 50, 51, 58
Drosophila, 14, 36, 42, 43, 106
drug therapy, 118
dysplasia, 61, 79, 82, 86

E

egg, 88
Egypt, 53
electrophoresis, 130, 132, 143, 154, 160
elongation, 16
embryogenesis, 21
embryonic stem cells, 43, 47, 86
employment, vii, 1
enamel, 102, 126
encoding, 17, 49, 61
endangered, 100
endocrine, 68, 113
endocrinology, 42
endonuclease, 145
England, 150
enlargement, 97, 100
environment(s), xii, 54, 67, 80, 121, 152, 158, 161
enzyme(s), 23, 145, 146
epididymis, 113
epigenetic modification, 29, 34, 49
epigenetic phenomenon, viii, 2, 32
epigenetics, 47
epithelium, 68
equipment, 121
erythrocytes, 21, 45, 147
ESD, 2
estrogen, 117
ethnic groups, 134
etiology, 115, 121
eukaryotic, 43, 97
Europe, 146
European Commission, 146
evidence, 9, 10, 11, 14, 15, 18, 19, 20, 22, 23, 24, 25, 26, 27, 45, 47, 48, 50, 77, 99, 101, 105, 112, 116, 127, 135, 153

evolution, vii, ix, 1, 2, 3, 6, 10, 11, 12, 18, 21, 32, 35, 36, 37, 38, 39, 40, 41, 43, 44, 46, 50, 51, 84, 88, 90, 92, 93, 94, 95, 98, 100, 101, 102, 104, 105, 106, 112
evolutionary history, vii, 1, 3, 10, 40
exclusion, 17, 105, 154, 159
exposure, x, 110, 118, 122, 142
extinction, viii, 87, 89, 100
extraction, 143

F

Fairbanks, 44
fallopian tubes, 117
false negative, 146
false positive, xi, 140, 142
families, 8, 12, 37
family history, xi, 139
family members, 136
female rat, 133
fertility, vii, viii, 13, 53, 54, 56, 58, 59, 62, 63, 64, 65, 71, 74, 75, 78, 85
fertilization, 55, 56, 69, 73, 75, 76, 88, 113
fetus, 65, 128, 130, 131, 141, 142, 143
fibroblast growth factor, 99
fibroblasts, 16, 22, 23, 46, 122
filtration, 143
fish, 17, 99, 106
fitness, 20
fluorescence, 10, 23, 99, 130, 138, 154, 160
follicle(s), 55, 66, 67, 68, 69, 76, 77, 99
force, 75, 96
forensic caseworks, x, 126, 133
formation, 11, 12, 33, 46, 62, 67, 75, 85, 90, 99, 113, 119
fragments, 126, 132, 134, 140, 143
fungi, 158
fusion, 6, 7, 10, 37, 94, 96, 97, 100, 105

G

gametogenesis, 9, 54, 56, 83
gel, 130, 132, 143, 154
gene amplification, 128

gene expression, 3, 12, 14, 18, 20, 22, 24, 25, 29, 30, 42, 45, 51, 63, 71, 72, 84, 106, 120, 123, 145
gene mapping, 7, 11, 37, 102
gene promoter, 30, 145
gene silencing, 18
genetic background, 57, 58, 59, 62, 64, 75, 123
genetic disorders, 141
genetic linkage, 37, 155
genetic marker, 127, 132, 158
genetics, 40, 42, 43, 46, 52, 77, 78, 81, 83, 101, 136, 153
genitals, x, 125, 127
genome, vii, viii, 1, 2, 3, 6, 7, 9, 10, 11, 13, 22, 26, 31, 37, 41, 78, 88, 96, 97
genomics, 5, 27, 101, 111, 161
genotype, x, 73, 82, 83, 125, 132, 162
genotyping, 149, 155
genus, 36, 79, 93, 94, 96, 97, 104
geographical origin, 133
Georgia, v, 139
germ cells, viii, 12, 15, 38, 50, 53, 54, 66, 74, 76, 77, 78, 81, 82, 85, 114, 115, 116, 118, 119, 120, 121, 122
germ line, 39, 77, 110, 111, 116
Germany, 154, 157, 158
gestation, xi, 83, 139, 140, 142, 144, 146, 148
gestational age, 144, 147
glucose, 45, 72
glycolysis, 72
gonadal dysgenesis, 76, 77, 85, 111, 114, 116, 117, 118, 119, 121, 122
gonadal microenvironment, x, 110, 118
gonadoblastoma (GB), ix, 109
gonads, vii, ix, x, 62, 65, 66, 77, 81, 82, 85, 89, 91, 92, 99, 109, 110, 115, 116, 117, 118, 119, 121, 122
grants, 75
Greece, 139
growth, 55, 67, 72, 77, 80
growth factor, 72, 80
guanine, 145
guilty, 153

H

hair, 57
hair loss, 57
haploid, 7, 12, 13, 15, 16, 54, 55, 60, 86, 88, 97
haplotypes, xi, 79, 130, 131, 136, 151, 153, 155, 157
health, 146
health services, 146
heterochromatin, 4, 30, 40, 47, 106, 111
heterogeneity, 160
histology, 116, 120
histone, 16, 29, 30, 31, 33, 34, 35, 43, 49, 50, 76
history, vii, 1, 3, 10, 40, 51, 157
homologous chromosomes, 11, 55, 66
hormone(s), 113
host, 111
human genome, 7, 37, 38, 44, 157
human remains, 129
humidity, 157
Hungary, 157
Hunter, 128
H-Y antigen, 111
hyaline, 117
hybrid, 34, 37
hybridization, 129
hydrocarbons, 158, 161
hyperandrogenism, 118
hyperplasia, 119
hypoplasia, 121
hypothesis, vii, 2, 5, 9, 11, 13, 15, 17, 19, 20, 21, 23, 28, 34, 35, 43, 48, 51, 60, 65, 75, 89, 99, 100, 105, 121, 122

I

ideal, xi, 54, 152, 159
identification, vii, xi, 10, 12, 57, 89, 91, 116, 127, 129, 132, 134, 136, 137, 138, 141, 149, 151, 152, 153, 158, 159, 160, 161
identity, xi, 151, 152, 154, 159, 160, 161
immune response, 111
immunofluorescence, 31
immunohistochemistry, ix, 109, 120
immunoprecipitation, 16
imprinting, 35, 51, 52, 56, 74
in situ hybridization, 10, 23, 99, 130
in utero, 3, 60
in vitro, 69, 70, 71, 76, 77
in vivo, 69
incidence, xi, 57, 83, 84, 118, 121, 126, 140, 141
incisor, 56, 80
incompatibility, 64
India, 130
Indians, 129
individuals, xii, 58, 117, 118, 129, 130, 134, 152, 159
induction, 119
industrialization, 153
inequality, 44
infants, 115, 135
infertility, viii, 9, 53, 54, 67, 71, 75, 115, 152
inheritance, xi, 73, 84, 88, 98, 100, 151, 152, 159
inherited disorder, 128
initiation, 16, 29, 42, 47, 52, 97
insertion, 133, 144, 149, 161
intact Y-chromosome, viii, 53, 54, 64
integration, 27, 99
intelligence, 9
interphase, 21, 70
intersex, 82, 98, 113, 128
intron, 10, 126
inversion, 56, 77, 88, 90, 105
invertebrates, 2, 10
Iran, 96, 136
islands, 30, 103
isolation, 96, 140, 146
Israel, 130
issues, 141
Italy, 64, 125, 134

J

Japan, 87, 94, 131, 151, 161

K

karyotype, ix, 39, 55, 62, 73, 78, 93, 96, 99, 106, 109, 114, 117, 121
karyotyping, 56
Kazakhstan, 96
kinetics, 104, 128
kinship, xi, 151, 152, 153, 155, 158, 159, 160
Kurds, 161

L

lactation, 3
lead, viii, x, 31, 61, 62, 87, 89, 100, 110, 116, 118, 122, 125, 126, 133, 143, 145
Leahy, 161
lesions, ix, 110, 115, 118, 120, 123
leukemia, 111
light, 44, 85
liver, 30
localization, ix, 23, 42, 48, 61, 65, 104, 110, 112
loci, xi, 23, 24, 31, 51, 99, 121, 129, 133, 134, 135, 151, 152, 154, 155, 156, 158, 159, 160, 161, 162
locus, vii, ix, 2, 5, 23, 27, 28, 31, 33, 47, 109, 126, 129, 130, 135, 136, 137, 155, 160
low risk, 122
lying, 25, 132
Lyon hypothesis, 21
lysine, 43, 49, 97
lysis, 143

M

machinery, 22, 28, 42
majority, xi, 32, 70, 91, 114, 139, 143, 159

Malaysia, 129
malignancy, 118
malignant tumors, 118
mammal, 26, 30, 39, 40, 103, 104
mammalian sex chromosomes, vii, 1, 5, 18, 35, 37, 40, 46, 107
man, 85, 105, 153
management, 123, 128
mapping, 3, 7, 36, 37, 99, 131, 159
marrow, 127
marsupial genome, vii, viii, 1, 2
mass, xii, 111, 127, 129, 152, 153, 159
materials, 55, 135, 153, 159
matrix, 126
matter, 44
MB, 129
measurement, 149
median, 16
mediastinum, 119
medicine, 152
meiosis, viii, 9, 10, 11, 15, 34, 52, 53, 54, 66, 67, 76, 77, 89, 90, 91, 97, 105, 110, 111, 155, 161
melting, 133
membranes, 51
memory, 48, 49
mental retardation, 9, 38, 98
messenger RNA, 41
meta-analysis, 144, 148
metabolism, 78
metaphase, 12, 30, 31, 70, 75, 84
methyl group, 145
methylation, 30, 31, 33, 34, 35, 43, 48, 49, 50, 145
Mexico, 75
mice, 21, 34, 47, 51, 56, 58, 62, 63, 64, 76, 77, 78, 79, 80, 81, 82, 83, 84, 85, 86, 91, 97, 99, 102, 105, 106, 122
microarray technology, 14
microRNA, 41
microsatellites, 153, 157, 162
microscope, 85
Middle East, 104
migration, 82
miscarriage, xi, 56, 139, 140, 141

Index

mitochondrial DNA, xi, 151, 153
mitosis, 21
model system, 42
models, viii, 10, 19, 35, 53, 54, 62
modifications, x, 14, 16, 23, 29, 30, 35, 43, 50, 110, 118
mole, ix, 88, 96, 104, 106
molecules, 141, 142, 143, 157
Mongolia, 96
monosomy, 115
Morocco, 157
morphogenesis, 113
morphology, 104, 120
mosaic, 42, 44, 55, 62, 111, 138
motif, 61, 84, 92, 101
MR, 135
MRI, 122
mRNA(s), 12, 41, 71, 86, 148
multiples, 10, 39
muscular dystrophy, 128, 141, 162
mutant, 56, 106, 122
mutation(s), viii, 5, 56, 57, 59, 61, 62, 77, 79, 81, 85, 86, 87, 89, 91, 99, 100, 102, 105, 106, 111, 114, 122, 126, 128, 129, 130, 134, 135, 137, 158, 161
mutation rate, 158, 161

N

National Academy of Sciences, 39, 41, 42, 43, 44, 48, 49, 50
natural selection, 9
negative effects, 72, 74
nematode, 14
neonates, 115
neoplasm, 116, 117
Nepal, 130
nested PCR, 143
non invasive prenatal diagnosis (NIPD), xi, 139
nondisjunction, 57, 81
nontumoral androgen-producing lesions, ix, 110, 115, 118
normal development, 54, 60, 61
Norway, 37

nuclei, 23, 30, 35, 41
nucleic acid, 147, 148
nucleolus, 30, 41
nucleotide sequence, 89
nucleus, 12, 70, 71, 73, 75, 112
null, x, 16, 62, 126, 129, 130, 131, 132
nutrients, 72

O

oocyte, viii, 53, 54, 55, 58, 60, 66, 67, 69, 70, 71, 72, 73, 74, 75, 76, 77, 83, 86, 113
oogenesis, 54, 56, 74, 77, 80
organ(s), 62, 127, 148, 154
organism, 19, 20
ovaries, 60, 64, 66, 68, 69, 71, 72, 76, 80, 85, 97, 99
overproduction, 142
oviduct, 113
ovulation, 69
oxygen, 72

P

pachytene, 11, 34, 41, 61, 66
pairing, 10, 11, 12, 41, 55, 61, 66, 85, 101, 105
Pakistan, 96
parallel, 37, 69, 70
parentage, 159
parentage analysis, 159
parents, xi, 152, 159
pathways, 24, 41, 104
PCR, x, xi, 22, 56, 71, 94, 99, 118, 125, 126, 127, 129, 130, 132, 133, 134, 136, 137, 138, 139, 141, 143, 144, 145, 146, 148, 149, 150, 152, 154, 158, 159, 160, 162
pedigree, 46, 153
penetrance, 62
perinatal, 60
peripheral blood, 115, 127, 136
perpetrators, 153
PGD, 122

phenotype(s), 21, 56, 57, 61, 66, 74, 82, 91, 106, 117, 126
phosphate, 45, 46
phylogenetic tree, 37
physical features, 140
placenta, 3, 22, 34, 38, 51, 141, 142, 145
plants, 10, 39, 110
PM, 123
point mutation, 61, 129, 134
polarity, 28
polyacrylamide, 132, 154
polymerase, x, 29, 43, 125, 130, 135, 141, 144, 149
polymerase chain reaction, x, 125, 130, 135, 141, 144, 149
polymorphism(s), vii, 22, 45, 46, 129, 130, 137, 147, 149, 155, 160, 161
population, x, xi, 21, 45, 93, 97, 100, 119, 120, 126, 129, 130, 131, 134, 135, 136, 137, 148, 151, 152, 159, 160, 161, 162
population group, x, 126, 129, 135, 159
population size, 93
preeclampsia, 141
pregnancy, 55, 56, 59, 77, 131, 140, 141, 143, 146
preparation, 143
preservation, 27, 76
prevention, 123
primate, 12, 13, 41, 42, 88, 100, 101, 122
probability, xii, 23, 152, 159
probe, 143
progesterone, 68
prognosis, 117
project, 22, 130
proliferation, 72
promoter, 14, 145
propagation, 26
prophase, 9, 41, 55, 60, 66, 67, 73, 76, 83, 105
prophylactic, 119
prostate cancer, 81
protein synthesis, 41, 55
proteins, 17, 26, 29, 34, 50, 52, 65, 66, 85, 102, 112
proto-oncogene, 116

prototype, 89

Q

quantification, 128, 133, 135, 141, 149
questioning, 15, 27

R

radiation, 7, 27, 30, 37
radiotherapy, 118
rape, 129
reactions, 143
reading, 65, 75, 91
reagents, 146
receptors, 69
reciprocal cross, 21, 34
reciprocal translocation, 10
recognition, 79
recombination, 5, 11, 12, 26, 32, 55, 82, 97, 100, 101, 110, 111, 129
recruiting, 26
recurrence, 118
red blood cells, 145
regression, 113, 114
rejection, 111
relatives, 110, 131
reliability, 150
remodelling, 25
replication, 21, 22, 30, 45, 48
repression, 12, 27, 29, 30, 34, 42
repressor, 25, 27
reproduction, 3, 9, 16, 36, 39
requirements, 120
researchers, 112, 130, 131, 142
resolution, 80, 131
response, 9, 19, 69
responsiveness, 29, 69
restriction enzyme, 146
restructuring, 37
RH, 138
risk(s), vii, ix, xi, 62, 109, 110, 114, 115, 116, 118, 119, 120, 121, 122, 123, 139, 140, 141, 142, 144, 146, 148, 162

Index

risk factors, 116, 120
RNA(s), vii, 2, 3, 10, 12, 15, 16, 17, 23, 24, 25, 29, 33, 41, 43, 46, 47, 48, 49, 50, 52, 86, 92, 121
rodents, ix, 12, 14, 18, 28, 34, 87, 103
Royal Society, 36, 38
rules, 26, 40

S

scholarship, 36
scrotal, 120
scrotum, 118, 120
segregation, 11, 12, 40, 60, 70, 77, 80, 98
seminal vesicle, 113
sensing, 25
sensitivity, 15, 20, 50, 116, 128, 143, 144, 146, 149, 159
sequencing, vii, 2, 3, 12, 15, 16, 22, 26, 27, 31, 43, 46, 50, 86, 92, 102, 150
Sertoli cells, 83, 112
serum, 128, 142, 147, 149
sex chromatin, 9, 21, 44, 45
sex ratio, 83
sex reversal, 51, 61, 62, 63, 64, 74, 77, 78, 79, 80, 81, 82, 83, 84, 86, 91, 99, 106, 121, 142
sexual development, 78, 84, 99, 116
short tandem repeat (STR), xi, 127, 151
showing, 4, 8, 13, 22, 38, 99, 129, 141
sibling, 37
signal transduction, 9
signaling pathway, 113
signals, 23, 80, 112
signs, 16, 76
silkworm, 17
silver, 154, 160
single X-chromosome, viii, 53, 56, 58, 60, 61, 66
skeletal remains, 127, 161
slaves, 105
society, 93
solution, 127
somatic cell, viii, 2, 20, 21, 23, 29, 53, 54, 63, 65, 72, 74, 77

South Africa, 106
South America, 79
Southern blot, 94, 99
SP, 109, 138
specialization, 9, 101
speciation, 38, 96
species, viii, 3, 5, 8, 11, 12, 13, 14, 18, 19, 22, 24, 26, 28, 30, 36, 37, 40, 41, 45, 46, 49, 74, 75, 87, 89, 91, 93, 94, 95, 96, 97, 98, 99, 100, 104, 105, 107, 112
sperm, 9, 13, 34, 38, 71, 93, 113
spermatocyte, 66
spermatogenesis, viii, 8, 9, 10, 12, 13, 38, 47, 51, 54, 57, 60, 87, 88, 89, 92, 96, 97, 102, 111
spindle, 69, 70, 72, 75
Sri Lanka, 129
stability, 30, 34, 74
stabilization, 30, 65
state(s), 17, 25, 29, 30, 43, 46
sterile, 63, 105
steroids, 69
storage, 71
stroma, 117
stromal cells, 120
STRs, xi, 130, 151, 153, 154, 158, 159, 160, 162
structural gene, 97
structure, 9, 11, 27, 38, 42, 63, 92, 103, 112, 113, 117, 126
subgroups, 122
substitution, 12, 91
substrates, 72
Sun, 138
supplementation, 70
suppression, 26, 28, 32, 88
surveillance, 61
survival, 36, 59, 67, 85
Sweden, 157
Switzerland, 64
syndrome, 38, 55, 61, 76, 79, 80, 85, 98, 101, 111, 114, 115, 119, 123, 124, 128
synthesis, 45, 49, 68, 114

T

tandem repeats, 152, 159, 160, 162
target, 13, 61, 89, 91, 112
techniques, vii, x, 1, 12, 125, 153
technology(s), vii, 2, 3, 31, 144
teeth, 157
telangiectasia, 122
temperature, 118
testing, xi, 126, 127, 131, 134, 140, 141, 146, 151, 152, 153, 154, 155, 158, 159, 160, 161
testis, ix, 5, 8, 9, 12, 13, 15, 16, 18, 32, 38, 41, 54, 62, 76, 77, 78, 81, 83, 89, 91, 92, 101, 102, 105, 109, 112, 113, 114, 115, 119, 120
testis-specific protein Y encoded (TSPY), ix, 109
testosterone, 68, 113, 117
thalassemia, 98
time frame, 30
TIR, 64
tissue, 12, 16, 24, 30, 34, 40, 60, 77, 120, 121, 136, 145
tooth, 92, 126
transactions, 36, 38
transcription, 13, 14, 16, 23, 25, 26, 27, 29, 30, 32, 34, 35, 42, 43, 55, 91, 98, 99, 112
transcription factors, 26, 29, 112
transcripts, 56, 81
transformation, 114, 118, 120, 121, 122
transfusion, 127
transgene, 29, 64, 78
translation, 31, 50, 97
translocation, 10, 47, 56, 97, 115, 118
transmission, 79
transplantation, 127, 136, 148
transport, 84
treatment, 142, 145, 148
triggers, 2, 25
tumor(s), vii, ix, 82, 85, 99, 109, 110, 111, 115, 116, 117, 118, 121, 122, 123, 127
tumor cells, 117
tumor development, vii, ix, 110
tumorigenesis, x, 110
tumours, 122, 123
Turkey, 96, 104
Turkmenistan, 96
Turner Syndrome (TS), ix, 110, 114

U

Ukraine, 96
ultrasonography, 140, 142
ultrasound, xi, 139, 140, 142, 146, 147
United, 39, 41, 42, 43, 44, 48, 49, 50, 134
United States, 39, 41, 42, 43, 44, 48, 49, 50, 134
USA, 79, 83, 84, 86, 106
uterus, 59, 99, 113, 117
Uzbekistan, 96

V

vagina, 113
Valencia, 67, 82
valgus, 115
validation, 146, 152
variations, 29, 31, 145, 152
vas deferens, 113
vertebrates, 12, 27, 37, 84, 105
victims, 161
visualization, 132

W

water, 157
West Africa, 135
World Trade Center, 161
worldwide, 157

X

X chromosome inactivation, vii, viii, 2, 14, 18, 20, 32, 33, 43-48, 50, 51, 52
X-chromosomal short tandem repeat (X-STR), xi, 151
X-inactivation, 28, 40, 44, 45, 46, 47, 48, 58

Y

yield, 149, 155, 158
Y-linked genes, viii, 87, 88, 89, 92, 93, 96, 97, 100, 102, 104
yolk, 51, 115, 116

young adults, 148

Z

zygote, 34, 55